PRAISE FOR
THE WORK OF
DR. ROBERT MELILLO

"A visionary new approach . . . These valuable clinical insights add much to our tool kit." —Daniel Goleman, author of *Emotional Intelligence*

"Clinically innovative and academically grounded . . . brings a refreshing, hopeful, and scientifically responsible approach to the field of childhood neurological disorders."
—Leslie Philipp Weiser, MPh, PhD, Harvard Medical School

"Whether ADHD, autism, dyslexia, or any number of neurobehavioral disorders affecting children, it is clear that what finally manifests represents the conspiracy of multiple events. As such, pursuing a multifaceted therapeutic approach as has been so deftly presented by Dr. Melillo offers up a welcomed and efficacious contrast to the myopia engendered in pharmaceutical mono therapy."
—David Perlmutter, MD, #1 *New York Times* bestselling author of *Grain Brain: The Surprising Truth About Wheat, Carbs, and Sugar— Your Brain's Silent Killers*

"Dr. Melillo is a true visionary in the area of childhood developmental disorders, and autism in particular. I have met with children and families whose lives have been transformed by his work. I know that his latest book will be another useful tool that will help others learn about and possibly prevent autism in their children in a way that only he can."
—Zac Brown, Grammy Award–winning musician, and founder of Camp Southern Ground

"Dr. Melillo's books are a ray of hope. Jam-packed with scientifically grounded information on brain function and its behavioral correlates, they provide satisfying explanations that parents recognize as relevant to their experience. And because his work is further tied to a simple intervention program, it has the power and potential to revolutionize the field."
—Michele Denize Strachan, MD, behavioral pediatrician, Developmental-Behavioral Pediatrics Program, University of Minnesota

continued . . .

"Dr. Robert Melillo is one of those rare individuals who can unravel the seemingly unsolvable mysteries of neurobehavioral development with wisdom, compassion, and vast perspective. His unique, groundbreaking, and research-based approach to improving brain function introduces the process of unlocking each child's potential."

—Pamela D. Garcy, PhD, clinical psychologist and professor of cognitive behavioral therapy, Argosy University, Dallas

"*Disconnected Kids* presents an optimistic and practical approach to opening windows of exploration, connection, and learning to all children. A highly recommended exploration for parents, educators, and therapists."

—Louis Cozolino, author of *Attachment-Based Teaching*

"Dr. Melillo, one of the world's leading experts in childhood developmental disorders, has organized the best scientifically referenced source of risk factors for autism, which all future parents should know about it. His book is a must-read."

—Datis Kharrazian, DC, DHSc, MS, MNeuroSci

"Dr. Melillo presents a very clear and educational view of how a child's brain grows, from the bottom up. . . . This is without any doubt an amazing theory that will stimulate a great number of research protocols."

—Dr. Calixto Machado, MD, PhD, FAAN, president of the Cuban Society of Clinical Neurophysiology

"Dr. Robert Melillo has unraveled the mysteries of brain organization and translated what we know into simple, practical therapeutic regimens to allow all of our children to reach their unlimited potential. He has produced a message of hope for parents of children, with clear, consistent, and significant results."

—Professor Gerry Leisman, director of the National Institute for Brain and Rehabilitation Sciences in Nazareth, Israel

THE DISCONNECTED KIDS NUTRITION PLAN

Proven Strategies to Enhance Learning and Focus for Children with
Autism, ADHD, Dyslexia, and Other Neurological Disorders

Dr. Robert Melillo

A TarcherPerigee Book

tarcherperigee

An imprint of Penguin Random House LLC
375 Hudson Street
New York, New York 10014

Copyright © 2016 by Robert Melillo, D.C.
Penguin supports copyright. Copyright fuels creativity, encourages diverse voices, promotes free speech, and creates a vibrant culture. Thank you for buying an authorized edition of this book and for complying with copyright laws by not reproducing, scanning, or distributing any part of it in any form without permission. You are supporting writers and allowing Penguin to continue to publish books for every reader.

Tarcher and Perigee are registered trademarks, and the colophon is a trademark of Penguin Random House LLC.

Most TarcherPerigee books are available at special quantity discounts for bulk purchases for sales promotions, premiums, fund-raising, and educational needs. Special books or book excerpts can also be created to fit specific needs. For details, write: SpecialMarkets@penguinrandomhouse.com.

Library of Congress Cataloging-in-Publication Data

Names: Melillo, Robert, author.
Title: The disconnected kids nutrition plan : proven strategies to enhance learning and focus for children with autism, ADHD, dyslexia, and other neurological disorders / Dr. Robert Melillo ; foreword by Zac Brown.
Description: New York, New York : TarcherPerigee, [2016] | Includes bibliographical references and index.
Identifiers: LCCN 2016003224 (print) | LCCN 2016007053 (ebook) | ISBN 9780399171789 (paperback) | ISBN 9780698170797 (ebook)
Subjects: LCSH: Pediatric neurology. | Brain-damaged children—Treatment. | Child mental health—Nutritional aspects. | BISAC: FAMILY & RELATIONSHIPS / Children with Special Needs. | HEALTH & FITNESS / Nutrition.
Classification: LCC RJ486 .M43 2016 (print) | LCC RJ486 (ebook) | DDC | 618.92/8—dc23

PRINTED IN THE UNITED STATES OF AMERICA

10 9 8 7 6 5 4 3

Book design by Spring Hoteling

Neither the publisher nor the author is engaged in rendering professional advice or services to the individual reader. The ideas, procedures, and suggestions contained in this book are not intended as a substitute for consulting with your physician. All matters regarding your health require medical supervision. Neither the author nor the publisher shall be liable or responsible for any loss or damage allegedly arising from any information or suggestion in this book.

The recipes contained in this book are to be followed exactly as written. The Publisher is not responsible for your specific health or allergy needs that may require medical supervision. The Publisher is not responsible for any adverse reactions to the recipes contained in this book.

While the author has made every effort to provide accurate telephone numbers and Internet addresses at the time of publication, neither the publisher nor the author assumes any responsibility for errors, or for changes that occur after publication. Further, publisher does not have any control over and does not assume any responsibility for author or third-party websites or their content.

To my beautiful wife, Carolyn. She is the best mom I know, and she has always promoted healthy food and a healthy lifestyle for our family. She has been my inspiration for all I have done.

CONTENTS

Foreword: Giving Back, by Zac Brown | ix

Zac and Me: How We Came to Be, by Dr. Robert Melillo | xiii

Introduction: Brain Imbalance and the Food Connection | xvii

PART I

BRAIN BALANCE NUTRITION: WHAT YOU NEED TO KNOW | 1

Chapter 1:
Inside the Brain of a Problem Eater | 3

Chapter 2:
Food Fight: Picky Eaters Versus Problem Feeders | 23

Chapter 3:
Searching for Food "Offenders" | 43

Chapter 4:
Feeding Without the Frenzy: Building a Healthy Relationship with Food | 69

Chapter 5:
Fueling Your Child with Brain Nutrition | 89

PART II

RECIPES FROM OUR STAFF AND GUEST CHEFS | 117

Chapter 6:
Start-Smart Breakfasts | 119

Chapter 7:
All Souped Up | 133

Chapter 8:
Dinner Delightful | 139

Chapter 9:
More Vegetables and Fruit, Please! | 165

Chapter 10:
No-Gluten Baking Your Whole Family Will Love | 181

Chapter 11:
Snacks That Don't Attack | 201

Acknowledgments | 217

Resources | 219

Selected References | 223

Index | 231

FOREWORD:
Giving Back

I learned a lot of things growing up in Georgia, but perhaps the most important lessons were those I learned at summer camp. I went to the kind of camp where special-needs kids were integrated into the environment with the rest of us, and it made an impression on me right from the start. I couldn't wait until I became of the age when I could return and work as a camp counselor—something I did for three consecutive years. The experience was invaluable. Watching the way kids from all walks of life can learn and grow together during just one week at camp is something that I've never forgotten.

For a lot of kids, going to camp and knowing they'll be able to come back the next year gives them something to look forward to all year long. They return home with a new perspective that builds character that lasts a lifetime. I remember that the children who arrived very shy and skeptical were often the ones who were crying at the end of the week because they had to leave their newfound friends and the counselors they had learned to admire.

Summer camp is especially meaningful for children with special needs. The integration process with mainstream kids through the daily activities that are part of camp life gives everyone involved a greater understanding of what these kids are living with day to day. Camp provides all kids with the opportunity to truly help one another and accomplish things that they never knew they could. Bonds are created within a group that inspire greatness. It helps prepare them for a brighter future and builds the confidence and security needed to play a productive and beneficial role in family and society.

I am a product of the camp environment, and it has changed my life. To have a place that is built especially for kids with specific disabilities with a staff that is sensitive to their daily needs would be a blessing to the children and their families. This has been my inspiration for Camp Southern Ground, a 400-acre state-of-the-art facility nestled in the farmlands of Fayetteville, Georgia, currently under construction and scheduled to open in the summer of 2016.

We are a camp whose purpose is to enrich and educate children with special needs and their entire families. Special-needs children require more than therapy. They need a lifestyle that is sensitive to how their bodies and brains function. This requires equipping the entire family with the skills they need to live to their healthiest potential. This is why health and nutrition are at the core of Camp Southern Ground—and why the Brain Balance Program is part of it. From our on-site organic farm to our farm-to-table education to our outdoor physical improvement opportunities, we will be able to help children learn how to take charge of their own health. These are lessons that cannot be learned soon enough. They are the lessons I have learned in my own life.

Finding the right balance among career, family, and philanthropy is always a moving target. A whole-foods diet and regular exercise not only make me feel better and more energized, they also ensure that I can be my best for the ones I love. I believe it is important to take care of our own selves well in order to lead a full life and have the energy to help others.

I have worked closely with Dr. Robert Melillo and the Brain Balance team for many years. I have seen firsthand the transformations in the lives of the children they serve. Brain Balance not only focuses on correcting their unique neurological challenges but emphasizes the whole health of each child—from their individual nutritional needs to their need for special daily activities to embracing and enhancing their family lives.

The missions of the Brain Balance Program and Camp Southern Ground create an undeniable synergy that will benefit the overall health of children with special needs. Brain Balance will be part of Camp Southern Ground and will help children with academic, social, and emotional difficulties reach their full potential and provide the tools necessary to achieve excellence in all facets of life. I am so proud to have Dr. Melillo and his team as part of our CSG family.

ZAC BROWN

APRIL 2016

ZAC AND ME:
How We Came to Be

Most people wouldn't imagine that a Grammy Award–winning, multi-platinum musician and a functional neurologist and expert on neurological disorders would have much in common professionally, but that's not the case with Zac Brown and me. We are finding that music and science mesh quite nicely when it comes to our mutual passion: helping children with special needs. As Zac says in his foreword, we have synergy and it is leading to great and wonderful things, most notably the creation of Camp Southern Ground and the Disconnected Kids Nutrition Plan.

Our remarkable kinship began in 2008, when our Brain Balance Program and the establishment of our Brain Balance Achievement Centers were really starting to take off. I got a call one day from Dr. Peter Scire, the co-owner and executive director of one of our first centers, Brain Balance of Greater Georgia in Peachtree City. He sounded quite excited as he told me he had met one of Atlanta's newest music sensations, Zac Brown of the Zac Brown Band, and that Zac wanted to come to the center to meet and talk to some of the kids and their parents firsthand. "He is really big in country music in Atlanta and is really interested in special needs kids," Peter told me. At the time Zac was a well-known local artist, but he had not yet released any songs or albums. Even then, however, his main passion was to develop a camp like the one he went to as a kid, which was for both typical and disabled kids. He immediately recognized the uniqueness of our Brain Balance approach and believed it might be something he could include in his camp that would help make it special. I thought, why not? and told Peter, by all means, to extend a welcome invitation. Zac sounded like a great person, and I was happy to help in any way. I didn't think much of it beyond that and went back to work. Little did I know back then that that call and the visit that was yet to be would inspire me to write this book—not just to help Brain Balance families but to also help Zac raise money to fulfill his dream of starting his camp.

A few weeks later I got another excited call from Peter. He had just taken Zac through the center and said the musician was very moved by what he had encountered. He had met children and their parents and heard remarkable stories of their transformation out of their diagnoses for such things as autism, Asperger's syndrome, ADHD, dyslexia, oppositional conduct disorder, and other disabilities. "Zac believes in our philosophy and what we are doing and said if we can help him with the development of his camp, he will do everything he can to help us spread the word about the work we do and our mission," said Peter. I have to admit that, being a born and raised New Yorker, I wasn't familiar with the Zac Brown Band and had only a passing interest in country music. I remember at the time thinking, *Well, that's really nice and very appreciated, but what could he do?* As it has turned out, he has done, and is still doing, *a lot.*

Zac's popularity started to skyrocket over the next few months after the release of his number-one hit "Chicken Fried" and a number of other hit singles that soon followed. In April 2009, after the release of my first book, *Disconnected Kids*, and soon after the release of Zac's first album, *The Foundation*, we had a chance to meet and talk on the eve of a book/CD signing that we were scheduled to do together in an Atlanta bookstore. It was the first time we really had a chance to get to know each other and share our stories and philosophies. We talked about his vision for the camp, why he was so passionate about making it happen, and our mutual vision of helping children with disabilities. I found out that Zac titled his first album *The Foundation* because it represented the charity he had started to raise money to build his camp. He told me the stories of his own days in summer camp and how he bunked with kids with autism and other disorders. He said his biggest dream was to open a summer camp for children with disabilities and that he had already purchased the land in rural Georgia. He told me of his vision for a big organic garden that the children could help tend and how they could be involved in the farm-to-table meals in a deluxe family dining center, where parents could also learn how to cook healthfully for their families. He talked about his dream for a state-of-the art aquatic center and lots of trails and open land where children could play. His goal, he said, was to make his camp special and unique in a way that would truly help transform children's lives. Brain Balance, he said, could be that conduit. As he spoke, his eyes lit up, and there was such passion in his voice, it almost moved me to tears. *This is a man with a mission*, I thought. *He's a doer. He's going to make all this happen.* I was committed to playing my part from that moment on. Later that evening at the book/CD signing, I gave a short talk, then introduced Zac Brown to the crowd. He stood up and started to talk and suddenly, in the middle of a sentence, his voice just cut off. I looked up and saw that he was so choked up with emotion, he could hardly get the words out. It wasn't the last time I would see that happen over this same topic. It was obvious to everyone that his passion for this subject was real and deep. Later, his wife, Shelly, told me she has rarely seen him choke up with emotion like that before.

I've learned a lot about Zac since that first time we met. He is a loving husband and devoted father of five—four girls and a boy. He also has another passion in life beyond his music and the camp—food. He just loves to cook for family and friends, and I can say from firsthand knowledge that he has quite the knack. If you follow the Zac Brown Band, you know that his Meet-and-Eat food fests prior to his shows are legendary, and if you've ever had the opportunity to attend one of these concerts, you also know the event is phenomenal. If you were listening closely between his songs, as I'm sure you were, most likely you also heard him speak of the Brain Balance Program and the work we are doing to improve the lives of tens of thousands of children. This kindness is not only helping to get the word out, as he promised he would do, but it already has had a direct impact on children, as you'll read in "A Mother's Story: Dear Zac" on page 11.

Not too long ago, my wife, Carolyn, and I had the chance to go along with Zac and Shelly to see the progress on the camp. It is amazing how far it has come since the first time we walked the woods together. What was originally intended to be around 70 acres is now several hundred acres in a new location that is even more beautiful than the original. As we walked the grounds, I was amazed by its beauty and all its greenery—and by how Zac could tick off the names of all the flowers and shrubs as we strolled on by. The facilities he is building are state of the art. The camp will be magnificent—there will be no other like it, and it will help thousands of children and their families. As Zac drove us back to the hotel, I couldn't help but tell him how thrilled I was that he took the time to show us his land and how honored I was to play a part in his dream. And, of course, the subject drifted to two of his other favorite topics: music and food.

"What's the connection?" I asked. "Why do you put the two together?"

"It's all about making people happy," he responded. "When it comes down to it, it is really all about love."

I couldn't agree more.

ROBERT MELILLO

APRIL 2016

Camp Southern Ground is a not-for-profit state-of-the-art facility in a bucolic setting near Fayetteville, Georgia, where both typical and special-needs children will be able to learn, play, prosper, and grow together. As of this writing, more than two-thirds of the $100 million needed to complete the camp has been raised from private donations. My proceeds from this book will be going toward the camp. For more information about the camp or to make a donation, go to campsouthernground.org.

INTRODUCTION
Brain Imbalance and the Food Connection

The Disconnected Kids Nutrition Plan is the natural follow-up to my groundbreaking book *Disconnected Kids*, which presented evidence that the childhood neurological conditions we know as autism spectrum disorder, attention deficit/hyperactive disorder (ADHD), dyslexia, processing and learning disorders, and the like all stem from one problem: an imbalance in the way a child's brain is developing. There is even a term to describe it: Functional Disconnection Syndrome, or FDS. The book explains in layperson's language how a myriad of these neurological conditions are really one and the same—FDS.

A functional disconnection is essentially a communication breakdown between the two hemispheres of the brain and areas within them caused by a developmental delay in one or both sides of the brain. The only thing that labels them as autism or Asperger's or oppositional conduct disorder (just to name a few) is the difference in their symptoms and which side of the brain is most affected. The book was first published in 2009, and a revised and updated edition was released in 2015.

Disconnected Kids was groundbreaking because it introduced the world to a new way to look at and treat these conditions through a holistic multimodal program I call Brain Balance, which addresses and targets what is actually going on in the brain. This had never been done before. Since we opened our first Brain Balance Achievement Center in 1994, we have expanded to more than one hundred locations all over the United States and have successfully helped more than 20,000 children. It's an astounding statistic, you might say, because many of these conditions—most notably autism—are still considered untreatable. But that is simply not the case. Scores of studies, including ones conducted independently on the Brain Balance Program and detailed in the revised and updated edition of *Disconnected Kids*, are proving otherwise.

THE PROOF IS IN OUR RESULTS

Even with the thousands of successes we have experienced in Brain Balance and its ongoing scientific scrutiny, the traditional approach by mainstream medicine continues to be medications or intervention programs that attempt to merely mediate the symptoms of such disorders rather than address the underlying problem—that is, what is actually going on inside the brain. Brain Balance was the first, and is still the only, program to do so. We have documented clinical evidence from thousands of children who have been through the program showing that it is possible to take a child who is learning below his age and grade level and bring him up as much as four levels or more after just three months on the program, and much more than that if children continue on the program for six or more months. We have also seen significant improvements in behavior and social interaction. In the same time frame, many Brain Balance children who had been professionally diagnosed as being on the autism spectrum or having ADHD, leaning disabilities, oppositional defiant disorder (ODD), dyslexia, and other conditions, can lose their diagnoses entirely after going through our program. While most of the children who come into our program are on medication, the vast majority are taken off of it by their own medical doctors after they complete the program because medication is no longer necessary. This is all because we address what is going on in the brain—a slowly or too rapidly developing left or right hemisphere, or in some cases, a slow-growing whole brain. As the two sides get back into balance, the symptoms significantly disappear or, as happens in many cases, go away altogether.

Prior to Brain Balance, no one had ever considered these conditions to be the result of what is happening in the brain. The idea of curing the problem was considered inconceivable—after all, many leading "experts" still believe that most of these problems, most notably autism, are being caused by some as-yet-undiscovered biological flaw. However, not one genetic mutation has ever been discovered that results in autism, ADHD, dyslexia, Asperger's, OCD, or the like. And I'm betting it never will.

Ask almost any parent who has been touched by autism or any professional involved in treating it what caused the problem and you'll most likely get a quick response: "It's genetic; you have to live with it." Some who are more attuned to what is actually being discovered by science these days might add, "It's environmental"—a truth I presented in my third book, *Autism: The Scientific Truth About Preventing, Diagnosing, and Treating Autism Spectrum Disorders—and What Parents Can Do Now.* When I give talks to parents and professionals, however, I always ask the audience a different question: "What is happening in the brain of someone with autism or ADHD or any of the neurological conditions we are seeing in children today?" I have yet to see a hand raised to answer *this* question. The truth is, the typical professional or clinician today still has no idea what is happening in the brain that is preventing a child from being able to learn. I think we can all agree that it is very hard to change a problem when you don't actually know what the problem is. Yet if you speak to any top brain researcher today, he or she will agree that the main problem in all of these disorders has to do with "functional connectivity" and that certain areas of the brain are not "talking" to or communicating with one another. I call that a functional disconnection and it is what makes the Brain Balance Program, including the at-home version offered in *Disconnected Kids,* so different from anything else being offered today. It is designed to get the two sides of the brain communicating again.

Brain Balance approaches the disorders that fall under the umbrella term of functional disconnection through a series of cognitive, academic, sensory, and motor exercises that can speed up a side of the brain that is growing too slowly or slow down a hemisphere that is growing too fast. It also provides a nutritional program designed to correct food sensitivities and an immature digestive system, which are part and parcel of a brain imbalance.

Only when the two hemispheres are functionally connected and in sync can the brain work properly and reach its maximum potential. An out-of-sync brain slows down or muddles the communication between the two sides of the brain, just as static on the radio makes listening impossible when it's out of range from the signal. This is why the problem is called a functional disconnect. For example, when a child with a functional disconnect reads a story, it's hard for her to follow along, because reading the words, a skill that resides on the left side, can't sync up properly and quickly enough with comprehension, which is handled on the right side. A brain imbalance can even bypass a needed skill altogether, which is why a child can seem indifferent or distant, lack empathy, be unusually clumsy, or act out inappropriately for no apparent reason. Simply put, the brain never quite got it together. The result is the classic unevenness of skills we see in all children with FDS, where they are much better than average or even advanced at certain skills and much worse or severely delayed in others.

THE GENETIC CONNECTION

How does this happen? This is where genes come in, but it has nothing to do with defects or mutations. Yes, there most certainly is a genetic link to all of the neurological problems we are seeing today, but it has to do with gene *expression*. The genes responsible for building the brain are either being turned on "off schedule" or are not being turned on at all. This is what science calls an *epigenetic effect*. There are more than 25,000 genes in the human genome, and 85 percent of them are believed to be responsible for building the brain and the billions of functional connections that make neuronal communication possible.

The human brain builds in a precise rhythm—mostly on the right side in the womb and from birth until around age two to three when it switches to the left, and then back and forth thereafter. When these genes are not turned on as scheduled, or when they're not turned on at all, the result can be a developmental delay on one side of the brain. The new learning that should have been put in place never happens. One misstep is not enough to cause a problem, but if the misses start to pile up, a gap begins to build that gets so exaggerated that it creates an imbalance—a functional disconnect. It's a sign of a combination of delayed or immature skills on one side and more advanced or exceptional skills on the other.

Gene expression is not automatic; it takes environmental stimulation—the kind that affects all the senses—to make it happen. Light, sound, taste, smell, touch, and especially gravity are all conduits of stimulation. If a brain is not exposed to environmental stimulation to turn on these genes at the right frequency at the right time, then growth is interrupted. The brain will be immature relative to a child's age. This does not mean that the brain is physically damaged; it just means the two sides are growing out of sync. A right-brain deficiency—the kind that causes autism, ADHD, Tourette's syndrome, or oppositional conduct disorder, for instance—is most common because brain growth is most vulnerable in the womb and early infancy.

Our environment today is a lot different than it was twenty, thirty, or forty years ago, which helps explain why the neurodevelopmental problems we are seeing now are *all* rising at epidemic proportions. Toxins in our air and water, sensitivities to heavy metals, an increase in Caesarean births and other birth traumas, overzealous use of sunscreen causing vitamin D deficiency, sedentary lifestyles, obesity, stress, and older men and women conceiving children, especially for the first time, are just some of the factors that have been linked to an increased risk of some of these conditions. In fact, studies have identified at least three dozen environmental factors linked to an increased risk of autism alone, and new ones are being discovered all the time.

NUTRITION AND THE BRAIN

The brain is like the CEO of human existence. It governs everything that happens in the body, and that means a brain imbalance affects every bodily system. It's why we see a myriad of subtle and not-so-subtle troubles in these children—from learning difficulties, social withdrawal, and out-of-control behavior, to chronic illnesses and inflammation, a heightened stress response, a compromised immune system, and poor digestion. We have found that an immature digestive system plagues at least 85 percent of children with FDS. They have what is called *leaky gut syn-*

drome, which means they can't absorb much of the nutrition from what they eat. And that puts them at risk for nutritional deficiencies. In fact, it puts them in double jeopardy because they aren't getting the essential nutrients needed to help the brain grow.

In the twenty-plus years that I've been working with children with FDS, I've heard over and over again from parents that one of their most perplexing and exasperating dilemmas is getting their child to eat right. Virtually all kids are fussy eaters, but kids with FDS are notoriously finicky. Parents are continually worried about their kids' nutritional status and their obstinate relationship with food. They're stressed over their inability—no matter how hard they try and how many fights ensue—to get their kids to eat healthily—or, in some cases, to eat at all.

Most kids with FDS have food issues. This largely stems from impairments in one or more of the senses. For example, a poor sense of smell can cause a disinterest in food, and an overactive sense of smell can make many foods repugnant. A child can be oversensitive to the tastes and textures of certain foods, which can make almost anything unappealing. For the most part, these kids start out life as difficult eaters and typically develop a liking for only a short list of foods—for many, a very short list. There is documented evidence in the scientific literature about children with autism who will eat only one food. It's as if they're addicted to a certain food or foods, which, you'll learn, they actually are! This frightens parents, and for good reason. A restricted diet in and of itself means kids can't possibly be getting the proper nutrition to fuel brain and body. The result is that many parents are spending thousands of dollars on special diets and foods, nutritional supplements, blood tests, and doctor visits in an effort to curb their child's dietary dilemmas. They are mostly told that their child has an immune system problem or digestive problem, that they have toxins in their bodies, or they may have vitamin, mineral, and amino acid deficiencies. In many cases, certain treatments lead to improvement, but they don't solve the problem. However, parents also are never told *why* any or all of these things are occurring—why their child has these nutritional, dietary, or immune issues, or why they have cognitive, emotional, motor, or sensory problems. The problems remain a mystery. Because they don't know what the actual primary problem is, parents continue to spend more time and money putting out fires and not dealing with the root cause. I can tell you, however, that all of these problems *are not* just one big coincidence: They are all connected to one another.

This is why I created the *The Disconnected Kids Nutrition Plan*. It is a complete at-home nutritional program designed to deliver optimum brain nutrition to children with FDS and steer them on course to a life of healthy eating habits. It is also designed to help parents offset the dinnertime dilemmas and food challenges that typically are part of everyday life. I need to caution you, though: It is not intended to be a singular approach to correcting a brain imbalance. If you have a child with FDS, you can follow the advice in this book to a tee, but your child is not going to realize his or her full potential unless you follow the motor, sensory, and neuro-academic exercises detailed in *Disconnected Kids*. For optimum results, a nutrition program should be initiated at the same time you start these exercises. This is not to say that you will not benefit should you follow this nutrition plan alone. While the best results from implementing dietary change will come from combining it with all other aspects of the Brain Balance Program—and it *is* what I recommend—many studies suggests you can still see improvement from the recommendations you'll find in this book, particularly when it comes to behavior issues, concentration, and focus.

As with all my other books, the information you'll find in *The Disconnected Kids Nutrition Plan* is a simplified version of what we do in our Brain Balance Achievement Centers, though it is designed to achieve results when followed properly at home. The nutrition plan we use in our centers is quite sophisticated and is customized to the individual child. This book offers parents solid information in a format that is neither intimidating nor overwhelming. Any parent should be able to follow the advice.

Though this book focuses on children with neurological disorders, it is of value to *all* parents because it addresses an important issue every one of us faces: getting our children the necessary nutrition to grow a healthy brain. That is what makes this book important to *all* families with growing children and why the advice and recommendations in this book extend to every member of the family.

It comes as no surprise to all caring parents that the food habits and practices adopted early in life are instilled for a lifetime. The challenge to instill them, however, can take on mammoth proportions when you have a child with a brain imbalance, and the fallout from a finicky eater can reverberate throughout the entire household.

This is not to discourage you. Quite the contrary. The problems you are seeing today—the fussiness, the clenched teeth, the unrelenting food fights that disrupt almost every family meal—will all go away as the brain gets back into balance with the Brain Balance Program. Your child may not be the perfect scout around food, but he or she will be no fussier than the next kid.

There is another reason you'll want to keep this book around. The recipes, nutritional plan, and practical advice found in these pages are designed to help nurture a brain all through childhood and into adulthood. The majority of the recipes were developed by mothers and fathers just like you—parents who have learned to deal with food sensitivities and the restrictions that go with them. When word got out to our Brain Balance families around the country that I was writing a nutrition and cookbook to help ameliorate the food issues related to a brain imbalance, I was overwhelmed by the generosity of so many parents who were willing to share their stories and offer the recipes their children enjoy. More generosity came from two extraordinary women—Donna Gordon-Teixeira and Jennifer Fugo—whom I met as guests on my television show, *The Doctor Rob Show*, which my wife, Carolyn, and I launched in 2013. Donna, a professional baker who now spends most of her time involved with Generation Rescue, the nonprofit national autism foundation founded by Jenny McCarthy, and Jennifer, founder of the website Gluten-Free School, generously offered to donate their professional recipes to the book for the benefit of Camp Southern Ground. Jordan S. Rubin, Ph.D., the dynamic founder of the leading-edge farm-to-consumer company Beyond Organic, contributed ten amazingly nutritious smoothie recipes featuring his products. My gratitude also goes to Christie Korth, Brain Balance corporate nutrition director and award-winning cookbook author, who has contributed recipes and has made sure all the recipes in the book foster good brain health. The contributions from all these dedicated people mean these are family recipes in the truest sense. Make them with love. When you fuel the brain, you also nurture the body. It means you're giving your child the best of both nutritional worlds. You can't do better than that.

PART I

Brain Balance Nutrition: What You Need to Know

Chapter 1
Inside the Brain of a Problem Eater

Imagine how you'd enjoy food if everything you ate tasted the same—or if you could barely taste it at all.

Eating isn't very exciting when all the senses are not engaged, and if you have a child with a neurodevelopmental disorder, he or she most likely also has some sensory issues—and that can make life at the dinner table quite traumatic as if you hadn't noticed!

In reality, your "picky eater" has a good reason for making a fuss around food, and a sensory issue is only part of it. As I explained in the Introduction, children with attention deficit/hyperactive disorder (ADHD), an autism spectrum disorder, dyslexia, a conduct or learning problem, or any of the other neurodevelopmental disorders listed on pages 5–6, share a host of social, behavioral, and academic problems related to the primary cause of their condition: a brain imbalance, or what we call functional disconnection syndrome (FDS). And when it comes to behavior, one commonality among virtually all of them is fussiness over food—in the extreme.

While you could safely say that most, if not all, children are fussy eaters, children with a brain imbalance are exceptionally finicky. For typical kids, their limited menu pretty much stems from the fact that their digestive system and taste buds are still maturing, and they have as yet to develop a palate for some of the stronger tastes that will appeal to them as they get older. But for kids with a brain imbalance, it's different. Many of them are not just fussy eaters, they're *problem feeders*.

Children with a brain imbalance have a battle with food that stems from a sensitivity in one or more of the senses. *All* the senses are involved in our appetite and appreciation for food—our *smell* (it can be anything from too powerful to nonexistent), our *vision (mmm, that looks good,* or *eeww, that looks yucky)*, our *touch (my son can't stand to even pick up the food in front of him)*, the *sounds (just the noise of a knife and fork seem to drive Billy to distraction)*, and, of course, the *taste (try a new food on my daughter— are you kidding me?!)*. Then there's *proprioception*, what we scientists like to call the sixth sense. It involves gravity—the way we feel our body in space *(I don't get it. Brenda continually fidgets and can't sit through an entire meal)*. Your child's response depends on whether he is *hyper*sensitive—too much of a good thing—or *hypo*sensitive to the point that the sense can be almost nonexistent.

At the same time, these children also have compromised or hyperactive digestive and immune systems. As a result, postmeal consequences can include any number of digestive upsets, from tearful bellyaches, to chronic constipation or frequent diarrhea, to gagging, reflux, and even daily vomiting. While to a parent this may seem to be just one more problem on top of autism, ADHD, or whatever, in reality digestive woes are part and parcel of having a neurodevelopmental disorder. The reason? It all stems from the brain.

THE BRAIN IS BOSS

The brain governs the body and all of the organ systems, so it only makes sense that a brain imbalance affects them all. The brain is in charge of everything—respiration, detoxification, the immune system, digestion, hormones, metabolism, you name it. All of these systems can operate without a brain, but they don't operate properly or optimally without the brain controlling and fine-tuning them. So, when the brain is out of balance, any, if not all, of these other systems will be affected. Numerous studies show that children with FDS commonly have chronic inflammation in the brain and body, a compromised immune system, and increased hormone levels due to a heightened stress response—the type of bodily turmoil that we do not feel but nevertheless exists around the clock. They also have lots of disturbances associated with digestion.

And, while learning the process of eating appears to be instinctive— a no-brainer, so to speak—it is actually one of the most complex skills a child needs to master, because it requires the cooperation of most of the body's organ systems. Swallowing alone involves the participation of 36 muscles and cranial nerves and the cooperation of the gastrointestinal tract and the vascular, endocrine, and respiratory systems. Both poor small-muscle control (indicative of a left-brain deficiency) or poor large-muscle control (a right-brain deficiency) will affect the ability to chew and swallow.

The fallout from this cascade of woes results in battles around food that are played out three times a day (or more), seven days a week. In the life of a child with FDS, this is pretty much routine. Your child is not being defiant, ornery, obstinate, or contrary on purpose. It's his brain imbalance that is making him act this way.

CONDITIONS THAT CAN BE IMPROVED

The following conditions fall under the umbrella term of functional disconnection syndrome (FDS). They have been shown to improve with the Brain Balance Program and can benefit from using the Brain Balance diet and nutrition plan. Throughout this book, all references to FDS apply to any of these conditions:

RIGHT-BRAIN DEFICIENCIES ARE DIAGNOSED AS:

- ADHD
- Autism and autism spectrum disorders, including pervasive developmental disorder (PDD)
- Asperger's syndrome, which is considered high-functioning autism and is on the spectrum
- Conduct disorder
- Obsessive-compulsive disorder (OCD)
- Oppositional defiant disorder (ODD)
- Non-verbal learning disability
- Tourette's syndrome

LEFT-BRAIN DEFICIENCIES ARE DIAGNOSED AS:

- Dyslexia
- Central auditory processing disorder
- Visual processing disorder
- Auditory processing disorder
- Dyspraxia
- Motor planning problems
- Learning disability
- Language disorder
- Reading disorder
- Sensory processing disorder
- Dyscalculia

POOR NUTRITION AND THE BRAIN

It is hardly a secret these days that the typical American diet is taking its toll on the health of our children (as well as adults) as evidenced by the rising rate of obesity and the earlier onset of serious but avoidable health threats, such as heart disease and diabetes. There hasn't been enough emphasis, however, on how poor eating habits are jeopardizing the development of a healthy brain.

Yes, you're probably thinking, you already know that the brain needs a steady supply of specific nutrients, notably glucose from complex carbohydrates, in order to function at optimum capacity. You probably know that proper nutrition supplies the raw materials needed for production of neurotransmitters, the chemical messengers that relay signals between the left and right hemispheres of the brain and beyond. You also know that we can think better and physically perform better after feeding the brain. And we've all seen evidence of how way too much sugar can turn kids into little monsters. But that's all old news.

What most parents don't realize is the detrimental effects a poor diet has on the developing brain, especially in children who already have FDS. It can have an impact on everything that is already troubling them—behavior, cognitive and/or academic achievement, sensory processing, gross and fine motor skills, equilibrium, immunity, and normal everyday bodily functions, such as digestion and elimination.

As I outlined in the Introduction, the developing brain needs a lot of stimulation from the environment, most notably in the form of movement, to flourish, but it also needs fuel. The brain's primary fuel supply is oxygen and glucose, which are manufactured during the digestive process from the nutrients in our food supply. A brain that has plenty of stimulation but too little fuel will not be able to take advantage of that stimulation.

Without fuel, the brain cannot make new proteins to build stronger neurons or make and repair cells that produce energy. Without fuel, brain cells will fatigue, get damaged, and die. Stimulation without fuel, or fuel without stimulation, simply does not work. Your child's brain can get all the stimulation in the world, but it will not be able to take full advantage of it without the right fuel in the right amount. Stimulation and fuel must work synergistically.

IS YOUR CHILD ON ADHD MEDS?

Ritalin and Adderal, two medications commonly prescribed for children with ADHD, can aggravate an already aggravating problem by killing the appetite. These drugs are stimulants that, like amphetamines, can dull the appetite to the point that your child will start losing weight. It's common for kids on one of these drugs to eat little during the school day until the drug wears off. Other side effects include abdominal pain, sleep disturbances, increased blood pressure, and inhibited growth.

If your child is on one of these drugs, you can help ward off the two major side effects—lack of hunger and sleep disturbances— by making sure he stays physically active throughout the day and keeps away from sedentary activities like computers, especially at night. Physical activity will help increase appetite and also help tire him out, so he will be able to fall asleep more easily.

Another reason to avoid computers and screens at night is because they emit blue light, which increases the production of cortisol and prevents the release of melatonin, which helps children fall asleep naturally.

I cannot emphasize enough how poor nutrition threatens the health of the developing brain, especially during the fast growth periods from infancy through about age three, when the brain grows from 25 percent to 90 percent of its adult size, and then again during adolescence, when the brain goes through another major growth spurt. Most children are fussy eaters, and exasperated parents will let them eat just about anything they want just so they eat *something*. However, this really isn't doing them much good in terms of their health. The National Academy of Sciences estimates that twelve million children get fewer nutrients than they need every day for optimum health. And it's not just poor food choices that are jeopardizing the nutritional status of our children. It's also what's in our modern food supply, or more to the point, what it lacks.

HOW BAD IS BAD?

Considering how much emphasis there is on food and the expanding American waistline, our dietary problems are only escalating. The problem isn't just what we are eating and feeding our children, it has a lot to do with what is and isn't in the food itself. The composition of the foods we typically eat—especially fruits, vegetables, and wheat—has changed tremendously, and mostly for the worse.

Farmed foods no longer provide the abundant nutrient levels that they supplied in the past. The rapid turnover of crops and overutilization of farming grounds continue to deplete minerals in the soil. According to one report, an average of 250 million tons of pesticides are used worldwide each year on crops that supply the fruits, vegetables, and grains we eat and feed to our children. This does not include the millions of tons of herbicides and fungicides used in the agricultural system.

Nonorganic food farms—which are, by far, the majority—feed hormones, antibiotics, and suboptimal feed to the cattle and livestock that end up on our plates. Soil, water, and air pollution continue to be major problems that affect everyone, but the toxic effects they have on children with brain imbalances can be quite profound.

In the last twenty-five to thirty years, food has become more and more processed, with tremendous increases in sugar, refined carbohydrates, and the worst kind of fats. Family dinners often consist of prepackaged meals too high in fat, artificial additives, and preservatives. And, of course, there is the keen interest among kids in consuming unhealthy soft drinks. Computerized records of the diets of one hundred children with ADHD, for example, found that sugary drinks frequently replaced milk at meals, snacks consisted almost exclusively of sugary or fatty foods, and fruits and vegetables were scarce.

EVEN THE WORST DIET IS NOT TO BLAME

I want to make one thing clear. A child's diet, no matter how poor it may be, does not cause autism, ADHD, conduct disorders, or any of the raft of neurological problems we are seeing today. The neurological problem, for the most part, has created a problem eater. Simply put, a brain imbalance compromises the immune and digestive systems that promote a cascade of digestive, intestinal, food, and nutritional issues that get played out every night at the dinner table. While it is highly unlikely that food is the source of the myriad issues that confront children with FDS, I do believe it can trigger and or exacerbate certain symptoms and can make the overall problem infinitely worse.

Meals purchased at fast-food restaurants are a common substitute for real meals, offering further nutritional depletion. These kinds of meals offer the lowest possible quality of ingredients, the most processing, and the two most common "vegetables" in too many kids' diets—French fries and ketchup! What's more, fast food is loaded with salt and saturated fat.

It's easy to see the negative effects such nutritionally empty foods can have on developing children. Study after study continues to support the link between poor nutritional habits and difficulties with focus, concentration, and attention in school and at home. It only stands to reason that nutritional shortages and toxic build-up will exacerbate the many difficulties associated with FDS, and it is happening in insidious ways that are finally starting to gain attention. Most notably, research now corroborates what we have been addressing in Brain Balance for twenty years: Children with neurodevelopmental disorders such as autism typically have immature gastrointestinal systems. This immaturity leads to an overactive "fight or flight" response by the sympathetic nervous system, which has major consequences on our digestive system. Research, including a paper recently published by me and my colleagues, has shown that kids with autism have an overactive sympathetic nervous system. At least 85 percent of the children who come through our Brain Balance Program have a digestive system that is dysfunctional in three primary ways. They have:

- Poor circulation and reduced blood flow in their intestines and stomach lining.
- Poor muscle tone and fewer contractions in the muscles of their intestines and stomach that help mechanically break down food.
- Less stomach acid and digestive enzymes, which chemically help break down food.

It all creates a vicious cycle that eventually leads to a condition called *leaky gut syndrome.*

A MOTHER'S STORY: DEAR ZAC
"Thank You for Saving Our Son"

This letter arrived at our Brain Balance Center in Atlanta with a request that it be forwarded to Zac Brown. It demonstrates the tremendous impact one generous gesture can have on the life of one child and his family. It moved me to tears and is an illustration of why Camp Southern Ground will be important to so many children.

Dear Zac,

My husband and I want to thank you for saving our son. Sounds dramatic, I know, but it's also very true. You see, not too long ago I attended one of the very best concerts of my life. I was blown away by your musicianship, by your gracious and appreciative manner onstage, by your letters for lyrics campaign, and finally (and most important) by the information you shared with the crowd about Brain Balance.

We have a beautiful little boy named Adam who sounded like a perfect candidate for the program you described. Adam just turned six years old and has a laundry list of medical issues including heavy-metal toxicity and numerous food allergies and sensitivities. He has a diagnosis of ADHD and sensory processing disorder. He is very easily overwhelmed by the sights and sounds of the world around him and has a tendency to be overly aggressive with peers and adults. He is also extremely smart, very loving, and laugh-out-loud funny. Until Brain Balance, these were qualities that were often overshadowed by his behavioral issues.

In order to truly appreciate how life-changing Brain Balance has been for Adam, you have to first understand what he has been through in the last three years. His dad and I are completely against drugging him into submission. We do not believe that the answers for Adam lie in signing him up for a lifetime of Ritalin or Adderall. We've tried meds for him—they don't work and almost always leave him in worse shape than when we started. And so we fight for him.

We had found Adam a wonderful naturopathic pediatrician, and the interventions we tried seemed to help until some infection or illness would set in and erase it all—until Brain Balance, that is!

After your show, I immediately ordered a copy of *Disconnected Kids*. Within the first two pages, I knew I was finally on the right track, and every page I turned made me even more certain that this program could help my son. I started the evaluation in the book myself, but called a Brain Balance Center in a town near me because I knew Adam needed help. He had just started kindergarten and was having a very rough time.

The center was able to create a home program for him and we began using it right away. We began seeing changes in Adam's behavior almost immediately, and within a couple of weeks, everyone else began noticing too. Less than four weeks into the program, he was making friends at school and bringing home happy faces from school! Adam still has a very long way to go, but his progress has been amazing, and we are completely confident that he *will* get there.

You have truly changed my son's life in all the best ways, and you have my eternal gratitude.

—Ally B.

BREEDING A VICIOUS CYCLE

When a baby is weaned from the breast and takes that first bite of strained carrots, pushes a soft cracker to her lips, or smashes chocolate cake around her mouth with her little fingers on her first birthday, it marks the true beginning of her lifelong relationship with food—one you hope will be spiced with love. And the digestive system is built to accommodate. As one new taste leads to the next, the digestive system naturally adjusts. As more food enters the mouth and goes down the hatch, it pumps more blood to keep the digestive processes moving. But when the digestive system is not maturing properly, this is not happening. A love-hate relationship begins instead.

Normally, the stomach is lined with closely linked cells that form a tight barrier from which only the smallest of molecules can escape. They form a protective shield against hostile invaders such as bacteria, viruses, fungi, and parasites that are seeking a place to breed. At the same time it is creating a properly balanced environment for the growth of good bacteria that is critical to good digestion and proper health. When blood isn't flowing properly, this protective seal becomes harder and harder to maintain. The stomach becomes vulnerable as the lining weakens, allowing larger molecules to escape into the bloodstream before they can be broken down to release important vitamins and minerals. At the same time, the stomach and digestive system gradually produce less acid and chemicals than are needed to break down food, absorb the nutrients, and create the proper pH balance. When food isn't broken down properly, important vitamins and minerals are not released into the bloodstream, meaning nutrients vital to the body and brain are lost. For instance, without acid in the stomach, we cannot absorb vitamin B-12 and folic acid, which are critical for proper gene expression. Many metabolic functions are affected as well, including brain development and function.

To complete the digestive cycle, food is broken down and moved into the intestines and bloodstream through a series of contractions known as *peristalsis*. When the digestive system is not mature, however, it produces these contractions less frequently, so food is not broken down adequately. It moves too slowly through the system, causing severe constipation, which eventually can lead to explosive diarrhea. This is the vicious cycle known as leaky gut syndrome. In fact in 2012, for the first time, the American Academy of Pediatrics conceded that "leaky gut" was real and that it is directly related to autism.

So even if your child's eating habits deserve a place on the honor roll, a leaky gut will prevent him from absorbing the precious nutrients needed during this time of vigorous growth, increased activity, and development of social and cognitive skills. Deficiencies in vital nutrients can compromise the full genetic potential of a child's mental developmental and physical growth. Virtually all kids with a brain imbalance have deficiencies in several important nutrients, and this can have a profound impact on behavior, learning, mood, and self-esteem. So, too, can another condition that is just as common in kids with a brain imbalance: food sensitivities.

BRAIN ALLERGIES, NOT FOOD ALLERGIES

When parents bring their children to one of our Brain Balance Achievement Centers for an evaluation, one of the first questions we ask them is: *Does your child have any food sensitivities?* Most immediately answer *no* and will argue that they'd know if their child has had a bad reaction to a certain food. Then I explain why they are mistaken.

Food *sensitivities*, often referred to as food *intolerances*, are not to be confused with food allergies. There is a big difference between the two. In fact, they bear no relationship to each other and even travel different immune-defending pathways.

Parents today know all about food allergies. These are the kinds of reactions in which a child eats a peanut or a piece of shellfish and within minutes, or maybe a few hours, will break out in hives, get watery eyes, start to sneeze, or even find it difficult to breathe. It can even result in life-threatening anaphylactic shock. This is the kind of allergy most parents live in fear of and are very cautious about. Only about 10 percent of children with a brain imbalance will have this type of allergy. However, more than 85 percent of them have food *sensitivities*—something that usually comes as a total surprise to their parents, especially when they learn that the foods their children are sensitive to are typically the kind of things they eat all the time.

The reason food sensitivities pass under the radar of even the most diligent parents, not to mention a lot of doctors, has to do with their insidious nature. They do not produce an allergic reaction that results in physical symptoms; rather, they produce an inflammatory response that results in more subtle mental and behavioral symptoms that can take anywhere from six hours to three days to appear. Research confirms that there is a direct correlation between this type of food sensitivity and an imbalance in the brain.

Food sensitivities and a leaky gut typically go hand in hand. The reason, again, has to do with the immune system. Most of the immune-system tissue that lines the gut—about 60 to 70 percent— protects it like soldiers guarding a fortress. It generally remains peaceable until it senses trouble. Then it'll jump into action and produce antibodies, which signal the release of inflammatory chemicals called cytokines, which call in white blood cells that pummel anything that gets in their way—like those large protein molecules that escape the gut. Like an allergy, it is an immune defense running amok.

It is important to understand that both allergies and food sensitivities are abnormal responses. For either to occur, two systems have to be functioning improperly—the digestive system and the immune system. And that always brings me back to the question: *why*? Why would both of these systems be dysfunctional? What is the link? The link is the brain and the overactive sympathetic nervous system. Ultimately, the brain is the cause or at least the major contributing factor, especially to a food sensitivity.

Unfortunately, when this happens often enough, the body becomes sensitive to these proteins and considers them enemies. Pasta after pasta after pasta at almost every meal looks like nothing but trouble. It's how kids with FDS end up with food sensitivities. Yes, that's right. The foods causing an issue for these children most typically are the foods they eat over and over and over again.

Unlike the obvious and often frightening physical symptoms of allergies, food sensitivities are difficult to identify because the symptoms appear gradually. These sensitivities do not produce the type of allergic response that we're all familiar with. Rather, they produce an inflammatory response with a completely different set of symptoms. Instead of the outward signs like a runny nose or watery eyes you might find with a mild allergic reaction, an inflammatory response will bring on behavioral, learning, emotional, and sleep issues. A parent would never suspect that their ADHD son's total meltdown at the supermarket checkout counter had a lot to do with the two slices of pizza he devoured at lunch *yesterday*. But it can and often will happen. Food sensitivities can only aggravate the actions and issues of children who already have developmental issues. These are among the symptoms that can be a sign that your child has food sensitivities:

- Aggressive behavior
- Bedwetting
- Chronic stuffy, itchy, or running nose
- Fatigue
- Irritability and total meltdowns
- Inability to focus or concentrate
- Impulsive actions
- Headaches, including migraines
- Hyperactivity
- Learning disabilities
- Mental sluggishness
- Muscle pain and soreness in the legs
- Pale, sallow complexion
- Puffiness or dark circles under the eyes
- Sleep disturbances, such as bad dreams and frequent awakening

IS YOUR CHILD ADDICTED TO PASTA?

If your child insists on eating the same food for dinner night after night, there might be an explanation for it: He or she could be addicted to it.

The vicious cycle that includes food sensitivities, poor digestion, and a leaky gut causes a cascade of chemical reactions, including the release of opiates, substances associated with addiction. This can actually make children crave the very foods that they are sensitive to.

I have found that most children with FDS will only eat certain foods. These foods generally contain dairy and/or wheat, including cereal and milk, cream cheese and bagels, macaroni and cheese, pizza, and pasta.

Normally, these foods are not problematic for typical children. In children with FDS, however, they cause a variety of negative effects and become almost like an additive drug. Likewise, a child can go through some minor withdrawal symptoms when these foods are eliminated from their diet.

A deficit in either side of the brain can lead to food sensitivities, though it is much more common in a right-brain dysfunction because this is the side of the brain that decreases the immune response and is responsible for decreasing the sensitivity of antibodies and reduces inflammation. With a right-brain deficit there is a relative increase in left-brain activity. This, in turn, increases the immune response and the sensitivity of the antibodies, causing the immune system to overreact and produce food and chemical sensitivites and inflammation. However, a deficit in either side raises the stress response and increases chronic inflammation, the primary catalysts for a leaky gut, which in turn leads to food sensitivities. As I've already noted, it is a cascade of events all caused by a brain imbalance.

A food sensitivity is more chronic, less obvious, and much more difficult to identify than a food allergy. People can, and do, live for decades without ever even knowing they have one. All they know is that they "aren't feeling right."

We'll get into more about food sensitivities and how to test for them in Chapter 3.

SEEKING PROFESSIONAL HELP

If you want or need professional guidance for your child's eating issues, seek the help of a functional neurologist, functional medicine specialist, or a nutritionist who has experience working with children with neurodevelopmental conditions. Functional neurology is a growing science and a field in complementary medicine that specializes in treating conditions through the brain-body connection. It is based on the philosophy that brain function and body processes are not totally integrated unless the brain is working as a whole.

If neither specialty is available to you in your area, take this book with you when you go to your first appointment with a nutritionist. It is imperative that the nutritionist understands the underlying causes of your child's brain imbalance and its nutritional repercussions.

To find a functional neurologist, go to IAFNR.org or functionalmedicine.org and click on "Find a Practitioner."

INFLAMING THE BRAIN: TOXIC BUILDUP

The immune response that goes hand in hand with a leaky gut and food sensitivities puts tremendous energy-depleting stress on a child's body—energy that is needed to build the brain. This produces another vicious cycle that I mentioned earlier—chronic inflammation.

Inflammation has several negative effects on the brain. It releases opiate-like chemicals that slow down processes and dull the brain, making a child appear to be in a fog. Inflammation also weakens the small muscles in the digestive system, making it sluggish and causing more constipation. When waste stays in the intestines too long, it begins to release toxins into the blood stream. This, in turn, puts more strain on the immune system and depletes the body's stores of natural detoxifying chemicals. This makes a child more vulnerable to the effects of mercury, lead, pesticides, and other toxic chemicals, all of which can harm both body and the brain. Inflammation can also challenge the delicate acid balance in the intestinal system, which contributes to the events leading to food sensitivities that I've already described.

All of this may start to sound overwhelming, but it is not too difficult to get these issues under control. In the next few chapters I will show you how to:

- Recognize the difference between a fussy eater and a problem feeder.
- Ameliorate some of the sensory issues that make for mealtime mayhem.
- Track down food sensitivities by putting your child on an elimination diet.
- Initiate strategies to bring mealtime harmony into your family life.
- Devise a supplement program that will help ensure that your child gets adequate amounts of the specific vitamins and minerals important to brain health. I will also explain why these nutrients are important to the brain and why they are particularly important to children with FDS.
- Make nutritious dishes that have passed the taste test of some of the most finicky eaters who have ever crossed the threshold of a Brain Balance Achievement Center.

DOES YOUR CHILD HAVE A BRAIN-RELATED EATING PROBLEM?

Central to the success of the Brain Balance Program is recalling the timing of important milestones from your child's early development. By extension, the same goes for getting to the root of your child's dysfunction around food. When a child has "blocks" in brain development, such as an exaggerated sense of smell or touch (hypersensitivity), we consider how this determines the child's relationship with food.

You should be able to find out if your child has an eating problem related to a brain imbalance by taking this simple test. The questions relate to developmental milestones specific to your child's eating habits until the age of two. If you have an older child, especially one who is ten or older, recalling these specific milestones might seem difficult. Answer these questions to the best of your ability. While you might feel it is hard to remember *exactly* when something occurred, I've found that parents most often can recall if something was amiss or didn't seem right. (To gain more insight into your child's developmental needs take the interactive Melillo 7-Day Challenge, which can be found at learn.drrobertmelillo.com/assessment/.)

It's best for each parent to take the test independently and then discuss your answers together. You may also want to involve a third party who may have been intimately involved in your child's care or upbringing during these years.

Please note: This test is not intended to be a diagnosis for a brain imbalance. Only a trained professional can ascertain for certain whether or not your child is developmentally delayed. Also, *Disconnected Kids* contains a Master Hemispheric Checklist and a variety of assessments to help you reach your own conclusions. If you have a child with a brain imbalance, however, this test will help you begin to unlock some of your child's behaviors and how they relate to food.

1. As a newborn, did it take your child 20 minutes or less to finish a 2-ounce bottle? (The average time is 5–20 minutes.)

    Answer: **Yes   No**

2. At 3 months of age, a baby should be able to take 20 continuous suckles from a bottle or breast without coming up for air. Breathing should follow sucking, with no pauses when she is hungry. Did your child follow this eating pattern?

    Answer: **Yes**   **No**

3. At 4 to 6 months, a child may still have a lingering tongue protrusion reflex. You would notice this if a child pushes food back out of his mouth while being spoon feed. It is a normal defense mechanism for an infant, but it is only normal up to 6 months of age. Did your child discontinue this "habit" by the age of 6 months?

    Answer: **Yes**   **No**

4. Some parents are instructed to give liquid to their children in a sippy cup around 6 months of age. However, some children are not ready for a sippy cup until 12 to 15 months of age, which is the normal age. Was your child drinking from a sippy cup by the age of 15 months?

    Answer: **Yes**   **No**

5. At age 6 months, a baby is ready to except thicker consistencies of food. Did your child begin eating baby food at age 6 months?

    Answer: **Yes**   **No**

6. By age 9 months, an infant should have started to munch on foods while eating, replicating the act of chewing. Did your child do this?

    Answer: **Yes**   **No**

7. By age 9 to 12 months, could your child eat without the support of a high chair?

    Answer: **Yes**   **No**

8. By age 9 to 12 months, did your child begin to take a controlled bite of a soft cookie, cracker, or wafer? If your child sucked on the cookie prior to biting, it was not a controlled bite.

    Answer: **Yes** **No**

9. By age 12 to 15 months, your child should have a well-coordinated suck/swallow/breathe sequence when given a spoon, meaning coughing and choking spells are rare at this point. Does this describe your child?

    Answer: **Yes** **No**

10. By age 12 to 15 months, was your child able to hold a baby cup with handles or a sippy unassisted?

    Answer: **Yes** **No**

11. By age 12 to 15 months, a child should be able to take a controlled bite of a hard cookie or wafer and have grasped hand-to-mouth coordination. Was your child able to feed himself a hard cookie at this age?

    Answer: **Yes** **No**

12. By age 2, a child should be eating a variety of foods from different food groups and with different textures, temperature, and tastes. Does this describe your child?

    Answer: **Yes** **No**

13. By age 2, a child should develop a sound style of eating and should be able to eat foods that are hard to chew, like meat and taffy. Does this describe your child?

    Answer: **Yes** **No**

If you answered "no" to four or more questions, your child most likely has a developmental delay that is affecting his dietary habits.

Chapter 2
Food Fight: Picky Eaters Versus Problem Feeders

If you have a child with an extreme sensory issue, you can bet a battle rages at the dining table pretty much three times a day every day of the year. These are not ordinary battles we're talking about where you're trying to talk your five-year-old out of requesting a waffle for breakfast, pizza for lunch, and pasta for dinner practically every single day. We're talking about a five-year-old who defiantly insists on eating the same thing *every* day at *every* meal and throws a fit if she doesn't get her way. That, in a nutshell, is what separates what we call picky eaters from problem feeders.

All parents can expect to see a certain amount of fussiness around food, especially when mom or dad sets something new on the dinner table—*ewww, what's that!?*—and expects everyone to just dig in. That's normal. However, if your child complains and resists trying virtually everything, then you might have a bigger problem on your hands. Here's how you can tell for sure:

Your child is a picky eater if she:

- Has a repertoire of thirty foods or fewer
- Wants to eat only certain foods for many days at a time
- Will switch to other foods and eat them over and over again, but will eventually want to go back to her former favorites after she's taken a break from them
- Doesn't like foods to touch one another on the plate
- Will not eat certain foods unless they are a certain temperature and/or consistency

Luke is a perfect example of a picky eater. Luke had just passed his first birthday when he started to display pickiness. Up until sixteen months of age or so, Luke ate all of his fruits, vegetables, and meat baby foods, without so much as a scuffle. In fact, Luke seemed to enjoy eating. However, when it came time to transition from stage-three baby food to table food, Luke found himself in distress. He began to turn down many foods, and this began to frustrate his mother. As a last resort, Mom decided to make Luke macaroni and cheese. Luke loved it and decided that is all he wanted to eat. Finally, when Luke became sick of mac and cheese, he moved on to something else and never really showed much interest in it again. But Luke was just going through a phase, just like any fussy kid.

On the other extreme, we have the problem feeder. Your child is a problem feeder if he:

- Has a repertoire of fewer than twenty foods
- Will eat only foods like deep-fried chicken fingers, hot dogs, pasta, and pizza and appears to be addicted to them
- Will begin to eat a food and will request only this food, eat it for several months, then switch to something else
- Has a strong phobic reaction to new foods and will often throw tantrums, scream, kick, and/or refuse to eat
- Rejects an entire food group, such as vegetables or fruits
- Does not want to touch food

Jack's story is quite different from Luke's. His mom can't remember a time when feeding was ever easy for her son. As an infant, Jack had a hard time with a bottle and would struggle to finish his meals. He also had a difficult time dealing with the transition from bottle to cup. At age five, it was not only that he was never hungry, his mom said, but that he didn't seem to enjoy eating at all. "It was almost as if Jack was afraid of food," she said. "Jack refused to eat any meat or vegetables." His disinterest in food had his mother frantic that he wasn't getting the proper nutrition he needed to grow and get his brain back in balance.

Jack is different from Luke because he had extreme sensory issues. Whenever kids have extreme sensory issues, it has a direct impact on how well they eat, their nutritional status, their early interest in food (which will help shape their future relationship with food), and, of course, what's going to get played out at mealtime in your household three times a day. While most kids with a brain imbalance are fussy eaters, about 60 percent of them are problem feeders.

PROBLEM FEEDERS AND FAULTY EATING MUSCLES

Problem feeders have a much more difficult time eating than kids who are simply picky eaters. One problem virtually all of them share is weak facial muscles.

When you think of kids with good motor skills, you think of kids climbing trees, playing hopscotch, and crawling all over the monkey bars at the playground. You never think about them chewing. Eating is a motor skill, however, and if a child has a problem with motor skills, as all children with brain imbalances do, they can also have a problem controlling the muscles in the face and mouth. And if they are having problems controlling the muscles in the face and mouth, they are going to be problem feeders.

Many people are unaware that we use the same muscles in the body to speak and eat. This is often the case in children with a right-hemisphere weakness. The right brain controls the large muscles and dictates muscle tone. This is especially true of children who are nonverbal. If a child is not speaking, then eating is surely going to be affected.

When a child's facial muscles are weakened by a brain imbalance, it can cause oral-motor skill delays that can make the act of eating physically difficult. About half of the problem feeders we see also have oral-motor skill issues, which are characterized by these symptoms:

- Loud gulping sounds when swallowing
- Coughing when trying to eat
- Appearing to choke when eating

- Gurgling when swallowing
- Looking distressed when eating
- Becoming fatigued as feeding progresses
- Getting watery eyes while eating or drinking
- Frequently refusing food
- Drooling mildly or heavily
- Having poor sleeping patterns, such as snoring and breathing through the mouth
- Having frequent illnesses, such as colds, coughs, and respiratory infections

It is no coincidence that a child who has an oral-motor weakness as well as speech and other problems also has issues such as autism, ADHD, or a learning disability. They are related to one another because they all are connected to the brain.

If your child is a problem feeder with any of these symptoms, you should see a speech therapist for an evaluation. A speech therapist can help correct the physical eating issues in a way that can work in conjunction with the Brain Balance Program.

EATING AND THE SENSORY-COMPROMISED CHILD

A hallmark of having a brain imbalance is having either an underactive or overactive sensory system: what we call *sensory processing disorder*. At least one of the senses will be affected, but we have found most children have problems with at least two or more of the senses. The most commonly affected are smell and taste. If you can't imagine what that's like, let me give you an idea:

Children with an underresponsive sensory system crave stimulation. These are the kids you see who like to spin in chairs, flap their arms, and act like the tough kid. They don't realize they're walking around with food on their faces. Eating isn't very exciting when all the senses aren't engaged, because these kids can't smell well and food doesn't taste like much of anything. But because their digestive systems aren't functioning properly, their bodies are craving nutrients, so they come across as ravenous eaters.

Despite their sensory issues, these children love to eat and can't seem to get enough food. Some of them surprise their parents by going for foods that are unusually spicy—more "grown-up" stuff like enchiladas or curries—because it gives them something they can actually taste. They enjoy exploring what's on their plates and can get so involved, they may find it difficult to move from one food to the next—eat the hot dog, then go to the baked beans, then the slaw; eat the chicken, then the fries. These are kids who can't seem to move away from their after-school snack to get back to their homework because they enjoy the stimulation they are receiving from the food so much. They tend to overeat because they lack the ability to feel full. They also have a tendency to overstuff their mouths for the same reason. About 45 percent of Brain Balance kids fall in this category.

At the other extreme, any kind of stimulation can be quite overwhelming for a child with an over-responsive sensory system. Tags on the back of clothing—and, in some kids, clothing itself—can be annoying. These kids can feel uncomfortable in even small crowds. Bright lights and loud noises can be extremely unsettling to them. Bring food into the picture—say a picnic or a barbecue—and they will become totally overwhelmed. The intense smell of food on top of all the noise and chaos is just too much for them. Instead of having a youngster who will want to run around and play and eat lots of fun junk food all day, you'll have a weepy kid who just wants to go home.

At home, these kids may avoid a food just because of the way it looks or feels. These are the kind of kids who may be willing to take a bite of something that looks inviting—*mmm, that bite of apple is mighty crunchy*—then spit it out a few seconds later when chewing starts to turn it mealy, a texture they just can't stand. Just the sight of eggs might sicken them to the point where they will start to gag, and if they'd dare take a taste, they'd probably throw up.

These are the kids who insist on eating the same foods day in and day out. Not only do they just want to eat chicken fingers and more chicken fingers, they insist on eating chicken fingers that come out of the same familiar box. Heaven forbid you mistakenly throw out the box and put the remaining morsels in another container because all heck will break loose—*Those aren't my chicken fingers!*

All children with a brain imbalance have imbalances in the sensory system that cause hyposensitivity to some stimulus and hypersensitivity to others. It is the nature of the imbalance. How they react to food—just how picky and fussy they'll be—depends on the severity of the imbalance. Sensory processing disorders or deficits are really sensory processing imbalances. For instance, a child with autism may be hyposensitive to low-frequency sounds, but may be hypersensitive to higher-frequency, louder sounds. This is not a sensory deficit; it is an imbalance.

If a child has a sensory processing disorder, here are some of the symptoms you are likely to see:

- Sensitivity to smells, temperature, and/or texture of foods
- Lack of awareness of flavor
- Difficulty manipulating eating utensils
- Variable attention during meals
- Dislike of the feeling of food or drink on the face
- Extreme sensitivity to the flavor of a food to the point that they are repulsed by it
- Frequent biting of fingers, tongue, or cheek while eating
- Inadvertent spilling of foods and drink, due to poor motor control
- Dribbling or drooling food down the cheek or chin due to poor motor control

By contrast, here is a food picture of what a child is like when his or her sensory motor skills are working properly:

- Can eat a nutritious meal from all four food groups without any trouble once transitioned to solids around age 1
- Can sit comfortably at a table and eat a meal with the family by age 4 or 5

- Can eat with utensils and has no trouble touching foods with hands at age 3 or 4
- Can eat food with peers and strangers by age 5
- Will be able to eat comfortably at a birthday party or any social function by age 5
- Can make friends and hold eye contact and engage in one-on-one conversation while eating by age 5

While the behaviors that define our sensory-compromised children appear erratic—and they are—to parents and observers, what you need to know is that they are not intentional. These children are not acting out and trying to destroy your mealtimes on purpose. They are not trying to be difficult.

THE CONSEQUENCES OF A LIMITED DIET

Delays in brain development change functions in certain areas of the brain that cause extreme sensitivity to the texture, smell, and taste of foods. Exaggerated perception of food texture can lead to avoidance of foods that have structural variations, such as broccoli. Children develop extreme sensitivities to smell because the pathways in their brains that perceive smells become overactive. In the case of broccoli, for example, it can then lead them to react to all foods rich in sulfur, such as onions, cabbage, and Brussels sprouts. A developmental delay can also lead to an inability to recognize taste perception efficiently, so a child may be attracted to sharp tastes such as extremely sugary foods or sharp cheeses, such as cheddar or blue cheese. This can lead to diets that are limited to a very small list of foods.

Unfortunately, this is bad news, because the diversity of the food we eat has an impact on the diversity of the bacteria species in our digestive system called *microbiota*. The microbiota is the ecology of microorganisms such as bacteria that we have in our intestines. Remember, we need to have healthy bacteria in our intestines, and recent research indicates that in order for us to be in optimal health, we need to have diverse species of bacteria in our digestive tract. The diversity of bacteria species that we have in our digestive tract is based on the diversity of our diet. So when we have a child who has limited his diet to only a few foods, such as pizza, sugary foods, and macaroni and cheese, we have very poor microbiota diversity. This leads to some major problems, including changes in brain functions such as mood, memory, focus, and concentration. There has been a surge of research in recent years on the gut-brain axis showing that the microbiota species in our digestive tract release neuropeptides and other cell messenger substances that have a direct impact on the brain. That's why it is essential that children with restricted diets learn how to eat healthily and diversify their foods with the strategies in this book.

. . . AND OTHER ISSUES

Resolving a sensory processing disorder, however, is imperative on a level greater than broadening a limited food repertoire and improving table manners. It's important because having a sensory issue also impedes a child's ability to respond to the world—to learn from it, to interact with it, to explore it. For example, let's take a look at just one slice of that universe: the world of food. Without a good capacity for smell, taste, touch, sight, and temperature, a child may not be able to visually identify an apple and a tomato or an apple from a tomato, a lemon and a lime or a lemon from a lime, or the temperature difference between a warm brownie and a bowl of ice cream. This means that in the future, such a child may have a problem developing a memory for food.

This is the case because identification and memory of things like food are more sensory processing skills then sensory detection skills. A child must first have the ability to detect food through sensory input before she can process and store it. One skill is built on the other. So if a child struggles with basic sensory detection of smell and taste, her ability to have higher-level processing of those sensory pathways is going to be compromised, delayed, or completely absent.

Although many practitioners will tell you that a sensory processing disorder is something that can be treated but not cured, we have found that sensory issues significantly improve or totally disappear in a large percentage of children who successfully complete the Brain Balance Program. As with all of their issues, a sensory processing disorder is just

TELLTALE TIPOFF OF A
FOOD AVERSION PROBLEM

Food aversion is an umbrella term we use for both picky eaters and problem feeders. In talking to parents at Brain Balance and hearing them describe the early feeding history they've had with their infants, we've seen a pattern that portends a future picky eater or problem feeder.

The quiz below will help provide further proof as to whether your child has a food aversion problem. Answer to the best of your knowledge. While it is often difficult to remember specifics from years past, we've found that parents do not have a hard time recalling if there were issues involved in feeding their baby.

- Did your child have difficulty bottle or breast feeding?
- Did your child have a problem latching on to the nipple or bottle?
- Did liquid or undigested food pour out of his or her mouth when feeding?
- Did you notice feedings were longer than 30 minutes?
- Did your baby make gulping or gurgling sounds while eating?
- Did your baby appear to become agitated while being fed?
- Did your baby's skin tend to turn red while being fed?
- Did your baby tend to have coughing fits during feeding?
- Did your child have trouble transitioning from bottle to cup and/or from liquid to solids?

If you answered "yes" to two of these questions, you likely have a picky eater. Three or more "yes" answers suggests a problem feeder.

another symptom of an undeveloped, unintegrated, and unbalanced brain. There is nothing broken in their brains, nothing "physically wrong" with the brains, and, in most cases, there is no pathology. It is not that these children can't detect or process sensory information at all. In most cases, they are hypersensitive to some sensory input and hypo-sensitive to others—they are unbalanced, just as their brains are unbal-anced. Resolve the brain imbalance, and the sensory issue should resolve itself as well.

In the interim, we have found there are measures you can take to help minimize the discomfort a child experiences going through these indi-vidual sensory issues. And in Chapter 4 we offer lots of solutions to im-prove life around the dinner table for your special child and the rest of the family.

MEALTIME SOLUTIONS FOR PROBLEMS WITH SMELL AND TASTE

If you had an overactive sense of smell—one in which odors were so strong that they repulsed you—it would pretty much be guaranteed that you wouldn't have much interest in food. Period. Why? Because if you can't stand the smell of something, you're not going to want to eat it. That's what life is like for a child with an overactive sense of smell.

Kids who have a sense of smell that is too strong can't stand the odor or taste of food almost to the point of repugnance. These are the kids you'll find holding their nose and running from the room, if not out of the house, if they smell broccoli or garlic cooking in the kitchen. Even foods as innocuously bland as bananas can smell like garbage to them. Sensitivity to odors can be so strong that some kids can smell what their parents are cooking for dinner while they're outside playing half a block away and come home complaining, *That's so disgusting!*

This kind of behavior is often quite puzzling to parents—and also quite frustrating—until they understand what's going on. On the surface, it ap-pears that their child is being overdramatic but in reality, to the child, the broccoli, garlic, or whatever is brewing in the pot really *is G-R-O-S-S!*

The health concerns that result from an oversensitive sense of smell go beyond food. Sensitive noses can smart against taking medications because of their noxious odor, even though the smell is undetectable to you, making family life even more exasperating.

Sometimes, more alarming to a parent is a little one who can't seem to be talked into eating *anything*—that would be a child with a *hypo*active olfactory system. But then would you feel like eating if everything tasted like cardboard? That's what it's like having an underactive sense of smell and taste.

An olfactory issue—either too much of a good thing or too little—is probably the number-one reason a child struggles with food. In my book *Disconnected Kids*, I describe a smell test using aromatherapy oils that you can give your child that will detect if his sense of smell is off and/or unbalanced. I also offer smell exercises that can improve, balance, and normalize the sense of smell and, by extension, taste. We have used this test and these exercises on tens of thousands of children in our centers, and 100 percent of them have shown objective measurable improvements to varying degrees in their sense of smell and in their processing of smell. Other than these activities, unfortunately, there isn't a whole lot you can do for a sensitive nose except keep foods as bland as possible for a hypersensitive child or perk up foods for a hyposensitive child. To help your child along until he or she successfully completes the smell exercises in *Disconnected Kids*, try the following:

Hypersensitivity

- Steer your child toward the blandest foods possible such as potatoes, rice, grains like millet and quinoa, corn, pasta, steamed vegetables, and plain chicken.
- Make ice pops from pureed fruits and vegetables, and try the assortment of smoothies in the recipe section. Freezing helps desensitize the palate, thus allowing a child the opportunity to try more foods.

Hyposensitivity

- Try adding strong spices to food—cinnamon, chiles, curry, turmeric, vanilla, etc.—and flavors such as onion, peanut butter, and almond butter to help stimulate the senses of taste and smell.

HOW TO EXPAND YOUR CHILD'S FOOD HORIZON

When parents have a child who is a fussy eater or problem feeder, especially when the problem is compounded by sensory issues, the thing they worry about most is whether their son or daughter is getting enough to eat.

Sure, kids like the taste of chicken nuggets (or whatever it is *your* child insists on), but it's much more than that. In their sensorily overloaded world, those chicken nuggets feel safe. It's what they know. Getting them to try something new is difficult because of the way their senses may respond—how those nuggets feel to touch, how they feel on the lips, the smell, the texture, the taste. Most kids with right-brain deficits such as ADHD, autism, and OCD don't transition to new things easily, and this includes new foods. That is because the left brain loves familiarity and the right brain loves novelty. The left brain, which is too strong in many of these children, is by nature obsessive and compulsive and wants to do the same thing over and over again. If the right brain is too weak, immature, or underdeveloped to inhibit the left brain, children become obsessive and compulsive about many things, including their food choices.

Christie Korth, Brain Balance corporate nutrition director, has coached hundreds of parents as well as other Brain Balance nutritionists on how to get the most finicky kids to try and like new foods. Here's what she recommends:

Start with an animated conversation about some foods your child would like to try. Make sure, though, that it leans toward something bland. Have them pick three: for example, a banana, chicken, and rice.

"Ask the child to inspect the foods," says Christie. "You want him to like it by appearance. Talk about it. Ask him what he likes about it, or what he doesn't like about it.

If he's engaged, ask him to pick it up and feel it. Talk about the shape, the color, the texture. How does it feel? Good or bad?"

If all's going well, the next step is to ask your child to bring it to his lips. "Ask what it feels like," says Christie. "Does it feel good or bad? If all's going well, the next step is to ask him to lick the food. How does it taste? Good or bad? Keep talking about the food, be encouraging." As long as the child is engaged and willing, even if he's a little hesitant but not reluctant, you can go to the next step: "Want to try to chew it?"

Always have a cup at the ready so the child can spit the food out, and a glass of water to get the taste out of his mouth.

The key throughout the entire process is to be totally engaging with the child through positive conversation. Give lots of praise as he passes through each stage. If at any time the child gets frightened or doesn't want to go on because he doesn't like the food, stop. On another day you can try some other food, but don't try the failed food until a month elapses. If your child ends up tasting the food and vomits, wait a full year before trying to reintroduce it.

Generally it takes trying a food ten to fourteen times before a child will take a liking to it. So the guideline here for the parent is: Be patient.

MEALTIME SOLUTIONS FOR SENSITIVITY TO TOUCH

Can you imagine a child who won't get near a hot dog or a hamburger? That might be a child with tactile issues—she is sensitive to touch. Such a child is so sensitive she doesn't like to touch food with her hands or will instinctively pull away when you put a plate of food in front of her. She might gag when touching food or, more likely, gag while eating.

This is also the child who can't stand the feel of food on her face—

like spaghetti sauce dribbling on the chin—and Mom constantly has to have napkins by her child's side so she can wipe her face and hands. At the other extreme, a hypotactile child will always be walking around with food on her face.

When it comes to touch and food, the brain can also send the taste buds mixed signals. For example, most kids go crazy for sprinkles on an ice cream cone, but not a kid with tactile issues. Just the idea of something crunchy like sprinkles on top of something smooth and soft like ice cream would be overwhelming and nauseating.

The concern for children with a hyperactive tactile system is that if they don't like the touch of food, they're not going to want to eat the food. They tend to play with their food as a way to stay engaged during mealtime and display indifference toward what's on their plate—acting as if all food tastes the same.

To give them an assist, here's what you can do:

- Designate and use food "mittens" so your child doesn't have to touch food at first. This can be an old pair of washable mittens that you can decorate for an eating occasion. A child is much more likely to take to something like this than to wear industrial food gloves, though you can give it a try.
- Introduce different textures of food for your child to touch gradually. If she likes soft (ice cream), then move to smooth (chicken), then go to bumpy (vegetables), then rough (nutty). Do it all by feel at first, without asking your child to eat the food. Once she gets comfortable with the feel, move on. This can help ease her out of her concern over the food.
- If your child does not tolerate the feel of food on her face, feed her foods that have a more dense consistency, so there is less of a chance of the food spilling on her face. For example, instead of feeding her sunny-side up eggs, try hard-boiled eggs. Opt for dense oatmeal and berries instead of cold cereal and milk.
- If your child is fussy about the texture of food and only tolerates, say, smooth foods, try to introduce other textures into

food gradually. For example, start with something soft, like rice or puddings, then advance up to nuts and seeds.
- Always have plenty of napkins on hand!

Disconnected Kids offers a checklist that will help you detect if your child is hypo- or hypersensitive to tactile sensations and processing. It also includes exercises that can help improve, normalize, and balance tactile sensations and processing.

MEALTIME SOLUTIONS FOR AUDITORY PROCESSING PROBLEMS

Remember what it's like being in the middle of a crowd in a packed stadium at a rock concert? Sensory overload—hands over the ears. That gives you an idea what it's like for a child with an auditory processing problem who approaches the dinner table with the television blaring in the background, dishes clattering on the table, siblings horsing around, chairs squealing across the floor, and everyone talking over one another. For a child with an auditory processing disorder, it's too much.

When there is too much noise going on around him, a child with sensitive ears will pay little or no attention to his food, which, as you know by now, presents its own set of problems. In order to stay focused and eat properly, he needs calm and quiet, with as few mealtime distractions as possible. Here's what you can do:

- Lower overhead lighting, turn off the television and radio, take the phone off the hook, etc. Doing so greatly increases a child's attention span and comfort throughout a meal, which, in turn, will help promote good digestion.
- For the same reasons, ban all screens from or near the dining table, such as cell phones, computers, and tablets.
- In-school lunchtime can be particularly hard on these children because the environment is typically anything but calm. Talk to the school and the person in charge of the lunch room about making sure your child sits in the area with the least noise and distraction.

- A noisy mealtime environment can be very distracting to a sensory-sensitive child, even if it seems normal to everybody else. People talking over one another can be very distracting and even confusing. One method we have parents employ that works very well is called the Talking Stick Method. The "talking stick" can be anything—a rag doll, a knotted piece of rope, a wooden spoon—that sits in a neutral part of the table at the start of the meal. No one can speak unless they have the talking stick in hand.

Disconnected Kids includes a checklist that will help you detect if your child is hypo- or hypersensitive to auditory sensations and processing. It also includes exercises to help improve, normalize, and balance auditory sensations and processing.

MEALTIME SOLUTIONS FOR VISUAL PROCESSING PROBLEMS

For a child with a visual processing disorder, the whole ritual around a meal—the table settings, the glasses, flatware, and the food itself—is so overwhelming it is difficult to focus on the food. If you have a child with a visual processing problem, you should approach mealtime like a minimalist:

- Limit place settings and flatware to only what's needed. Keep serving dishes on the kitchen counter, and plate the dishes in the kitchen or let family members serve themselves.
- Allow your child with the sensory issue to be the first to be seated. This allows him or her the opportunity to be at the table when it is at its least distracting.
- Keep your child's portions small. The smaller the size, the less visually distracting it will be. Encourage second helpings and even thirds.
- The color green is known to have a calming effect. Use a green tablecloth or placemats.
- Contrasting colors at the dinner table are also a great idea. For example, use a white plate with the green tablecloth or

placemat. A white plate will allow your child to easily distinguish the color and texture of each food. For example, green spinach and orange carrots will show up nicely on a white plate but not on a blue plate.

- Colored forks and spoons can also help your child visually process the foods on the white plate much better.
- Get rid of fluorescent lighting. This can be harsh for a child's eyes and can cause the child to zone out on the foods instead of eating them. Use natural lighting whenever possible.

Disconnected Kids includes a checklist that will help you detect if your child is hypo- or hypersensitive to visual sensations and processing. It also contains exercises that will help improve, normalize, and balance visual sensations and processing.

BRAIN BALANCE PROFILE
Stephanie Couldn't Sit Through a Meal

Stephanie's story illustrates how a weak vestibular system—the sense that gives us stability and allows us to feel grounded—can interfere with the dynamics of eating. Though Stephanie had a lot of behavior issues, most disruptive to her family was her inability to sit through a meal. No matter what her parents would do, how often they would coax, cajole, or even threaten, Stephanie could not sit at a meal for more than five minutes before getting up and running around the table or from room to room. Her urge to move her body was that strong. Round and round she'd go, meal after meal, day after day. "It's so bad," her mother told me, "it's impossible to take her out anywhere or to anybody's house to eat. We don't even like to take her to her grandparents' for dinner."

Stephanie was the classic example of a Disconnected Kid with a right-brain weakness. Her bad table manners were a side effect of poor proprioception—she didn't feel her own body very well, a sign that she had major issues with her vestibular system. While her family, especially her siblings, thought Stephanie was a mealtime problem, what they didn't realize was how distracting mealtime was for her. Because she came from a large family, the household tended to become loud around dinnertime, when homework was winding down and the television came on, dad was coming home from work, and activity was taking place in the kitchen. Stephanie's sensory system tended to be underactive, so running around helped stimulate her senses, which helped drive her oral-motor skills to eat.

In addition to the typical Brain Balance protocols we initiated—nutritional and supplement programs; motor, sensory, and neuro-academic exercises—we found the most noticeable difference came from the small interventions we used to deal with Stephanie's weak vestibular system.

For one, we found that Stephanie had a lingering primitive reflex called a spinal gallant, which was contributing to her inability to sit still at the dinner table, and we showed her parents a simple exercise that would take care of it. What seemed to really do the trick, however, was a simple contraption we devised: a special cushion with foot straps for her chair at the dining table. With her feet in the straps, she felt more stable and grounded. This made her feel safer and reduced her anxiety. She was no longer compelled to get up and run around during meals.

Six months later, her parents reported that Stephanie was sitting through complete meals without the compulsion to get up from the table. For the first time in as long as they could remember, they could finally take the family out for dinner.

IS YOUR CHILD A LITTLE SQUIRMER?

Proprioception, which is often referred to as our sixth sense, is related to gravity—our ability to feel ourselves in space. It's what makes us feel grounded. Kids with a brain imbalance often have poor proprioception. They have little or no perception of what their bodies feel like. Children who are not aware of their own bodies feel particularly anxious and unsafe in situations where there is a lot of sensory stimulation taking place. Mealtime, as you might imagine, is one of them. As a result, they can develop a conditioned negative response to mealtime and eating.

Many children with poor proprioception are squirmers—they just can't seem to sit still, something that becomes a point of distraction when the family sits down for a meal. As I touched on in the introductory quiz on page 19 in Chapter 1, this is most likely due to a lingering primitive reflex called the *spinal gallant*, which exists at birth to enable a newborn to travel through the birth canal. It is supposed to die out naturally at around four to six months of age. Lingering primitive reflexes are among the issues contributing to a brain imbalance, and that includes sensory issues. Having a lingering primitive reflex or reflexes is nothing to be alarmed about. People can go through life without ever completely getting rid of them. They are, however, easy to shed.

You can abate the spinal gallant through an easy-to-do exercise that is fun because it mimics the fun children experience when playing the game angels in the snow:

> Have your child lie face up on a mat or flat surface with his legs extended and arms at the side. Have him breathe in and simultaneously spread his legs outward and raise his arms out along the floor and overhead until his hands touch, as if he were playing angels in the snow. Have him exhale and return to the original position. Do this five times a day several times a day until the squirming stops.

Another way to help your child feel more grounded at the table is to put a step stool under her feet while eating. For children who are reluctant to sit at the table, try having a picnic with them on the living room floor.

MEDICAL CONCERNS AND FEEDING ISSUES

If your problem eater frequently or repeatedly displays any of the following symptoms, you should consult with your child's pediatrician. It's likely there is something more going on other than the symptoms and problems associated with being a problem feeder or having a brain imbalance. You may need to take your child to a specialist such as a gastroenterologist or an allergist.

- Bowel obstruction
- Choking when eating
- Colic
- Coughing
- Deficiency in one or more B vitamin
- Diarrhea
- Difficult or painful swallowing
- Gagging in response to food
- Food getting stuck in throat
- Heartburn
- Hives after eating certain foods
- Lack of appetite
- Noisy breathing
- Retching while eating
- Spitting up
- Vomiting or episodes of severe vomiting (known as *cyclic vomiting syndrome*)

Chapter 3
Searching for Food "Offenders"

"Food sensitivity" is likely to take on a whole new meaning when you embark on the venture of trying to find out which foods may be triggering some or all the erratic behavior you are seeing in your child with a neurodevelopmental disorder. That's because on this journey you must get your child, who already has a very limited diet, to give up his or her favorite foods. But here's the silver lining in this seemingly black cloud: It will only be temporary.

The process is called an *elimination diet*, and it has been around for decades. With all the advances we have made in modern medicine, no one has yet come up with a better way to detect a food sensitivity. While it is not fast, it is effective. Nutritionists use it routinely to get to the bottom of all sorts of puzzling dietary dilemmas.

Embarking on an elimination diet is challenging in and of itself, but it can be an especially daunting process when you have a child with a brain imbalance. Through our own clinical observations in our achievement centers around the country, we have seen the extreme lengths many children will go to in order to manipulate their parents to give them their favorite foods, even to the point of refusing to eat *anything* (though they eventually *do* eat). But our experience with tens of thousands of children is proof that it can be done, and I will show you how. First, let's get through the protocol, and then in the next chapter I will offer you some helpful tips the nutritionists and parents at our centers have found work— maybe not like magic, but pretty close. Yes, it is possible to remove *"I-want-my (fill in the blank)"* offending foods and gradually introduce a more healthful and varied menu into your child's life. I'm even going to go out on a limb and say the experience can be not only painless, but even I dare say fun for both you and your child.

THE 10 MOST WANTED LIST

A child can be sensitive to *any* food, but we've found that most children with neurodevelopmental issues have a problem with the same foods or ingredients. And again, it is not unusual for a child to have an intolerance to more than one food.

On the surface, the foods on this 10 Most Wanted list appear to have nothing in common and, in fact, may even surprise you because they are all nutritious. As you read through the list, think about your child's relationship with each food—does he love it or hate it? Just tuck that knowledge away in the back of your mind for the time being. You'll learn what to do with it soon enough. Here is the top-ten list, starting with the most common suspects:

1. Gluten

The word "gluten" defines a cluster of proteins found in certain grains, most notably wheat. A decade ago, practically no one knew what it was, let alone gave it much thought, except for the unfortunate less than 1 percent of the population who had celiac disease. Today we know that gluten is much more invasive and is the most common food sensitivity associated with a brain imbalance. Kids with a leaky gut cannot properly digest gluten, and the molecules can escape the gut, creating all kinds of stomach upsets. In addition to wheat, other common grains containing gluten are barley and rye. While oats traditionally do not contain gluten, they can be contaminated with it during processing.

2. Dairy Products

What, a child being sensitive to milk? But it's a major food group, right? Yes and yes are the unfortunate answers. The substance of interest is casein, a protein found in milk, including goat's milk.

Gluten and dairy are chemically very similar, so if your child has a problem with one, he most likely will have a problem with both. There are lots of different kinds of casein, and the one found in cow's and goat's milk is the most problematic. It is likely that your child could be sensitive to milk, for example, but be perfectly fine with certain types of cheese. This is why you need to treat milk and cheese separately on an elimination and rotation diet. A casein sensitivity should not be confused with lactose intolerance, which is a sensitivity to the sugar in milk. It is possible for a child to be sensitive to both casein and lactose.

3. Eggs

Eggs may be considered the perfect food—and were once unjustly accused of raising cholesterol—but they are imperfection in a lot of little tummies. The trouble with eggs is that they are mucous forming, and mucous is not well tolerated by a leaky gut. We may not think we eat a lot of them but we do, because they appear in so many foods, especially baked goods. And remember, sensitivities occur from eating the same foods over and over again. An egg sensitivity is almost as common as a sensitivity to gluten and casein. It should not be confused with an egg allergy, which produces an immediate reaction and is common in babies and young children.

4. Baker's and Brewer's Yeast

If your child has been exposed to a lot of antibiotics and has had a lot of yeast infections, he or she could have developed a sensitivity to the proteins found in baker's and brewer's yeast. Unfortunately, the list of foods containing yeast is huge and includes a large variety of commercially prepared products and baked goods.

5. Legumes (Beans and Peas)

We all know that beans are not easy to digest, even by the best of stomachs. So you can imagine the havoc they can cause to a leaky gut! The instigators are the sugars in the beans, which also make them so caloric. Green peas also fall in this category. A lot of kids would jump for joy over this one! Botanically, peas are a legume, but nutritionally we tend to view them as a green vegetable. The protein in peas is poorly digested.

EXCEPTIONS TO THE RULE

Chickpeas and peanut butter are two legume foods you need not be concerned about (as long as your child does not have a peanut allergy). They are more easily digested than other legumes. Chickpeas are great because they are the lowest of all the legumes in sugar. If you are going to feed your child peanut butter, make sure the peanut butter was processed from non-genetically modified peanuts and that it is labeled natural and organic.

6. Apples

What?! Whatever happened to an apple a day keeps the doctor away? Apples have chemicals called salicylates in them that are believed to lead to behavioral issues and hyperactivity in some children.

7. Tomatoes

When parents hear this one, they often say, *Yikes! My kid lives on ketchup and pizza.* And there is probably a good reason why. As you learned in Chapter 2, kids are most often sensitive to the foods they crave. It's like an addiction. Tomatoes are a common problem for a lot of people with sensitive stomachs because of their high acid content, and that includes little ones with leaky guts.

Taking tomatoes away from your child will not be as difficult as it sounds. In fact, when you get to the reintroduction phase of the elimination diet, we have a recipe for a healthier homemade version of ketchup from a Brain Balance consultant who found it cleared up a lot of issues with her ketchup-loving daughter.

8. Soy

Okay, so your child isn't going to go to bed crying because he can't have tofu for dinner or Tofutti for a Saturday-night treat. But if you depend on a lot of packaged foods in your household, soy is more prevalent in your child's diet than you may realize. The problem with soy is twofold: It is generally too processed, and it is abundant in too many processed foods—the reason your child could develop a sensitivity to it. Soy also contains phytoestrogens, and too much soy in the diet can raise estrogen levels, which have been implicated in other health issues.

9. Corn

Corn probably wouldn't have even made it on the list a few generations ago, but that's before the phrase *Genetically Modified Organism (GMO)* made its way into our nutritional lexicon. Corn is very poorly digested, which is why a leaky gut can't handle it. It is also very different than the corn our ancestors ate. Case in point: Back in the 1930s, a stalk of fresh summer corn contained 98 percent protein and 2 percent sugar. Today it is just the opposite: 98 percent sugar and 2 percent protein. We have been eating GMO corn since the 1970s.

THE GMO TRIUMVERATE

Wheat, soy, and corn are the most common GMO crops in our foods supply today. An estimated 99 percent of crops are believed to be in some way genetically modified. The only way to avoid them is to buy from organic farms.

10. Citrus

A sensitivity to citrus foods is another one parents have a hard time dealing with, because if there is one highly nutritious drink they can usually get their kids to swallow, it is orange juice—and, of course, less-nutritious lemonade. However, the high acid content of citrus is tough on a leaky gut, and a lot of the citrus drinks sold in the marketplace are really only disguised as "authentic" fruit juice. They can turn into double trouble because they can actually kill beneficial digestive enzymes. Even if your child is not sensitive to citrus, you're best off avoiding citrus juices and teaching your child to enjoy water as a beverage instead.

PLAYING FOOD DETECTIVE

As I've noted several times already, food sensitivities are not as easy to detect as food allergies. Consider that a good thing, because a sensitivity is not life threatening. However, their insidious nature of producing symptoms, mostly of the behavioral type, hours or even days later make them difficult to detect. One clue that can be considered a red alert for possible food sensitivity is erratic behavior. This is the kind of behavior in which your child is good as an angel one day and the exact opposite the next. Or perhaps your child is acting quite normally, and then about an hour or so after a meal, all heck breaks loose. Or the child has meltdowns every day around the same time, and that happens to be two hours after lunch or breakfast. If your child is eating the same foods every day and is having meltdowns around the same time of the day, then food or sleep issues, or both, are probably to blame. Wild swings of this type are a tip-off that you will most likely find a culprit when you do the elimination diet.

It *is* possible to identify a food sensitivity on your own. The difficulty comes from the process you have to go through to get there. I won't sugarcoat it; it can be tedious, but it can go smoothly if you are diligent and patient. The entire process will take about a month. This procedure is going to help you identify:

- If your child is reacting to a specific food and if that reaction is responsible for some of the behavior you've been seeing
- Which specific symptoms may be related to which specific foods
- The severity of the reaction
- If your child will benefit from eliminating a certain food from his diet
- How to design the diet

FOOD AND THE FAMILY

A food sensitivity, just like a brain imbalance, may not fall far from the family tree. The only difference between you and your child is the severity of the problem. For you, the same food issues may be or may have been so mild as to be barely detectable. Or, put another way, you may have or may have had a brain imbalance too.

I pointed out how this can happen in my book *Autism: The Scientific Truth About Preventing, Diagnosing, and Treating Autism Spectrum Disorders—and What Parents Can Do Now*. Scientifically, it's called an *epigenetic effect*, and it is the most logical explanation for linking genetics to autism or any of the other neurodevelopmental disorders discussed in this book.

In a nutshell, epigenetics means that there are factors, mostly in the environment, that can affect if and when certain genes are expressed. For example, numerous studies have documented the presence of autistic symptoms or traits, ranging from mild to severe, in the close relatives of children with autism. It is even possible that mild traits of food sensitivities or a brain imbalance displayed themselves in ancestors you may not even know existed, gradually became more pronounced through the generations to your grandparents, to your parents, then to you, which resulted in a full-blown sensitivity in your child.

While food sensitivities tend to run in families, the reason you are seeing them with all the severity your child can muster is most likely because other developmental issues associated with a brain imbalance are making them worse. For instance, you may have been a very picky eater when you were a child, but now you have a child who is truly a problem feeder. You may have been a highly active child, but your child has full blown ADHD. The basic genetic trait has always been there, but the severity has to do with the level of gene expression. This is epigenetics. The good news is that it is changeable.

Step 1: Do the Detective Work (7 to 10 Days)

This is the most important part of the process. For the next week to ten days, you will do nothing different with your child's diet except keep track of everything she eats. It is important to not stray from the norm. This is not the time to introduce new foods or recipes!

Get a notebook or use your computer and write everything down—every morsel your child eats, how much she eats, and the time of the day she eats it. Arrange your notebook by meal and snacks. If you use prepackaged, canned, or frozen foods, keep the packages, as you will want to check the ingredient lists to see if any of the ingredients appear to be causing a reaction. This is very important because prepackaged foods contain a lot of offending ingredients and chemicals. Soy, for example, shows up in some of the most unlikely places.

In addition to recording all foods eaten, you will also write down all the behavioral or other out-of-the-norm symptoms your child displays throughout the day. Note the time of day and how long the symptom lasts. Remember, sensitivities generally bring on behavioral symptoms hours or even days after a problem food is eaten. If you've written it down, you can look back to see if you can detect a pattern of food and behavior.

This task is a lot easier if you are totally in control of all meals, so do it at a time that makes this possible, such as during a school vacation. If this is not possible, make sure you prepare your child's school lunch and away-from-home snacks. Make sure your child brings home his lunch pack with any uneaten food, so you can record accordingly. Stress the importance of not trading lunch and quiz him every day after school about what he ate while away from home. If your child spends time with a caregiver, fill her in on what you are doing and enlist her help in tracking these events. Stress the importance. Also inform your child's teacher about what you are doing. While you can't expect a teacher to keep your log for you, you can ask her to tell you about any behavioral issues as they arise.

Step 2: Round Up the Food Suspects

After a week or so, you should have a bona fide record of your child's eating *and* behavior patterns. Now, this step is equally as important as Step 1, but it is more challenging than your fact-finding mission because you are going to have to come up with some assumptions. Like any good detective, review the facts. Pore through your notebook looking for patterns between foods eaten and subsequent behaviors. Keep in mind that there could be a big time lapse between the two—several hours or even a day or two. For example, if Joey eats pizza a couple of times a week for lunch and throws a whammy a few hours later, then has pasta and sauce for dinner and starts to give his sister noogies while she's trying to do homework afterward, then tomatoes might turn up as a suspect. But don't forget the wheat (gluten) in the crust and pasta. Both should make the list. Look for a pattern.

Does some unflattering behavior usually show up some time after chili night? Then it's a pattern. Or maybe you serve tacos every Friday night and you're wondering why every Saturday afternoon with little Sarah is an exercise in defiance. Could there be a relationship between the behavior and the corn tortillas? Possibly. That's a pattern. Add corn to the list. But what else do you put in those tacos? Investigate—maybe it's the salsa. Could it be the tomatoes? And what about the citrus that goes into it too? If you see a pattern, add it to your list. Do you see other behavioral issues emerge after your child ingests an orange or orange juice? If other citrus products don't show up later in a behavior issue, you know it's not the citrus in the salsa creating the problem. Scratch it from your list.

In every instance, err on the side of caution. If something strikes you as "not so sure," then put it on the list. You'll learn soon enough if it's safe to add it back into the diet. Do not be concerned if you have ten or more foods on your list. This is quite common.

Because wheat (gluten) and dairy (casein) are the most common food sensitivities in children with FDS, you should consider them your chief suspects. These two foods are also chemically very similar, so it is likely that if you discover one to be a problem, the other could be as well. I generally tell all parents to start out eliminating gluten and casein on the elimination diet, even if you don't suspect they are causing overt symptoms, because they are such common sensitivities these days. It is entirely possible that you will find no patterns between your child's food choices and his behavior.

A DIFFERENT KIND OF BEHAVIOR PROBLEM

Not all children with a brain balance are troubled by food sensitivities, though the majority are, especially children with a right-brain weakness. It is also possible that your child has neither a food sensitivity issue nor a brain imbalance. The problem simply could be a behavior problem, though "simply" is not the choicest word. How to arrive at this conclusion and what steps you can take to handle it are all covered in my second book, *Reconnected Kids: Help Your Child Achieve Physical, Mental, and Emotional Balance.*

Step 3: Take Them Out of Circulation (4-plus Weeks)

This is where the, *ahem*, fun begins. This is when you will eliminate all the suspected foods from your child's diet, but rather than do it cold turkey, which is what a typical elimination diet recommends, we suggest doing it gradually.

Introducing a transition period makes it a whole lot easier, especially for a child who has to give up a food that is like an addiction. It means you can ease away from the physical dependency and at the same time start to gradually introduce and experiment with better, healthier substitutes. For example, swap out cow's milk and substitute almond, coconut, or another nut milk. This will make the withdrawal much more manageable than going cold turkey. Also, by the time you get to full transition, your family will be better prepared. You might already start to see changes in behavior or even an improvement in grades. If this is the case, you definitely know you're on the right track!

This stage is the best part because it marks the start of something I consider to be bigger and better: the beginning of a new lifestyle of healthy eating for your entire family.

Yes, to be most effective, the entire family has to be involved in the process, and that includes Mom and Dad. One reason is that you can't eventually start depriving Johnny of some or all of his favorite foods and expect him to go along with it willingly if he has to go solo. You don't want to hear a lot of *Why can Brian have Wheaties and milk and not me?* Talk about battles around the kitchen table! If Johnny has to switch to Rice Krispies and almond milk, then Brian should, too, and Mom and Dad as well.

The other reason, which you'll learn more about in the next chapter, is that you want to establish a dinnertime discipline in which the entire family is served the same thing. This doesn't mean you can't pack different lunches for your kids, if you don't mind and it helps your sanity, or that all family members can't fend for themselves at breakfast, if this is the best thing for your lifestyle. But when the family sits down to eat a meal together, it should be the same meal. This is especially crucial when you are eliminating gluten, casein, eggs, and or any of the other foods that showed up on your list. You don't want your child to feel singled out and have to watch others eat what he can't have. You'll only have misery on your hands.

It is so easy to put a positive spin on this. It is the perfect opportunity to get your family to start eating more nutritiously and to establish healthy eating habits. Tell your family it's an experiment for *all* family members as part of your new goal to eat more healthily. It's also the ideal time because the foods on your chief suspect list are not the only things that you must exclude on an elimination diet. For the next four weeks you must also eliminate:

- Junk food—this means all fast food, candy, pastries, soft drinks, etc.
- Processed foods—this includes deli meats and cheeses and most fast-to-the-table foods that come packaged
- Food additives—this requires checking labels carefully. The list of food additives is long, and you should familiarize yourself with them. As your cheat sheet, consider anything off limits that contains these words: agent(s), enhancer, regulator, gums, and anything ending with 'ant.'

You should expect a little mayhem at first, especially from the child who is the focus of this exercise. You'll be expunging all these foods for four weeks because you want to make sure to get them all out of his system. As I've already mentioned, kids can crave the foods they are sensitive to, like addicts. And, as with an addiction, you can expect some withdrawal symptoms. If you have gradually reduced these foods, then this withdrawal may be less severe, but even so, your child may experience any or all of these common symptoms for about the first two weeks:

- Irritability
- Depression
- Lethargy
- Difficulty sleeping

Keep in mind that the more severe the withdrawal symptoms, the more the child needs to be on this elimination diet and the more improvement you will see later on.

When the diet is done correctly, these symptoms will disappear before the month's end and you will see a significant improvement in general health and behavior. If not, it means one of the following:

- Your child cheated and ate off-limit foods without your knowledge.
- You have not properly identified the food or foods your child is sensitive to.

- Your child does not have a food sensitivity.
- You did not follow the steps of the diet properly.

It also means you can't move on to the next step. You'll have to go back to Step 1 and start all over again. So before you get started, reread these steps carefully, be diligent in your detective work, and rigid with the rules. It's that important!

THE ELIMINATION DIET MADE EASIER

Virtually every child who has ever gone through the Brain Balance Program has also gone through the elimination diet described here, and that includes tens of thousands of kids. No one knows better than our Brain Balance nutritionists and the parents who have put their child or children through the program how challenging a task it is—surmountable, yes, but challenging. For you, however, we're going to make it much easier.

These same people who have "been through it all" were more than eager to share their experiences with you by offering the sensitive-foods-free recipes they made and are still making for their families. Part II contains nearly one hundred recipes—all taste-tested by kids, including some of the most finicky eaters we've ever met. All the recipes are gluten free and virtually all are free of casein. With a few exceptions, these dishes avoid all the foods on our 10 Most Wanted List. Recipes that do contain one of these food suspects have footnotes. You can make the recipe without the ingredient or save it until you start reintroducing this food back into the diet.

We love these recipes and trust you will too.

Step 4: Reintroduce the Food Offenders

Proceed to this step only if Steps 1 through 3 have resulted in a noticeable improvement and after your child has been off the offending food for at least thirty days. You will now begin to reintroduce back into the diet the foods that you have isolated for suspected food sensitivities. You will reintroduce them one at a time, but the order in which you do so does not matter.

If your child has a right-brain deficiency, I recommend that you begin this process on a Saturday. Children with a right-brain imbalance generally act out more over the weekend. For kids with a left-brain imbalance, behavior issues are typically more noticeable during the week, usually around homework time. For them, begin this step on a Monday.

Again, you will use your notebook and record every meal, with emphasis on the food that is being reintroduced, and follow these instructions:

- First thing in the morning, make a note of the quality of sleep your child had the night before and your child's general demeanor throughout the day. For example, is he listless, moody? Does he have a stuffy nose? Any changes for the better or worse in any area, including sleep patterns, can be considered a negative reaction to a food or foods, so it is important to be aware of all of these functions. Take note of them. On the day you reintroduce a new food, serve it at breakfast, lunch, and dinner and increase the amount with each meal.
- It does not matter which food you start with, although you should reintroduce milk separately from other dairy foods.
- Record the quantity of the food eaten and the time.
- As you did before, look for behavioral symptoms or any significant changes in the child's overall health and demeanor and record them—what happened, when it occurred, and how long it lasted.
- Reintroduce the food for only one day and remove it again from the diet, even if it does not produce any symptoms.

- On days 2 and 3, keep all the suspected foods out of your child's diet, just as you did in Step 3. It may take up to three days for negative symptoms to appear, so pay close attention even on the third day. If symptoms arise, it means the child is sensitive to the food and should not be eating it at all or until her brain becomes more balanced. Wait for all symptoms to disappear before reintroducing the next food. If there are no food reactions at all, then proceed to the next food.
- On day 4, reintroduce a second suspected food back into the diet, following the same process as described above. As with the first food, the following two days should be clean days in which no suspected foods are eaten.

Follow the same process one food at a time until all the foods on your list have been reintroduced for one day. If your child gets sick during this step, suspend the process until after recovery.

Now here's the most important part: If at any point a reintroduced food produces symptoms, it is a sign that your child has a sensitivity to this food. If this happens, suspend what you are doing until all the symptoms disappear and are gone for a full twenty-four hours. Then continue on with the other foods on your list.

Step 5: Come to the Conclusion

If your child has a food sensitivity, you will see a clear pattern develop in which certain symptoms will develop after a certain food or foods are eaten and then subside after the foods are removed again from the diet. Consider these to be foods to which your child is sensitive and remove them completely from your child's diet.

I have found this to be an excellent and accurate gauge for finding the foods a child is sensitive to. If you feel you need confirmation, however, ask your child's physician to do a standard blood test called an IgG food intolerance test. IgG stands for immunoglobulin G, one of the five subclasses of antibodies the immune system releases to chase specific antigens. (Food allergies occur on a different pathway called IgE). The test can confirm if your child is sensitive to a specific food.

If your child is following the elimination diet in conjunction with the Brain Balance Program, it's likely you may see the behaviors you spotted in Step 1 diminish by the time you get to this level. Consider this a good thing because it is a sign that the Brain Balance exercises that you initiated along with the nutritional portion of the program are starting to take effect.

GETTING BACK TO NORMAL: THE ROTATION DIET

A rotation diet is much like Step 4 of the elimination diet but is a more formal approach—one that factors in a total nutritional approach that guarantees your entire family will take advantage of *all* food groups. You can start a rotation diet when your child is ready for you to begin reintroducing the foods he or she has been avoiding; that is, when all the behavioral symptoms he was displaying have disappeared or have significantly dissipated and you see improvements in other areas of life that are the hallmarks of a brain imbalance—notably the cognitive, sensory, and motor issues that I touched on in my Introduction and detailed in *Disconnected Kids*. As you see improvement in these areas, you'll see improvements in your child's digestive and other related problems as well. That means his food sensitivities will fade away too.

This is when you can start thinking about getting life back to normal and start to bring these foods back into your child's life again. By *normal*, however, I do not mean the *I only want chicken fingers and ketchup* of the past, but a new normal of a variety of highly nutritious foods that are good for the brain and body.

This does not mean your child can never have chicken fingers and ketchup again—in fact, we offer several versions of healthier chicken fingers in our recipe section. You'll find lots of the healthier versions of many of your kid's favorite foods, especially sweets and snacks. And they're all gluten free, so you won't have to worry about loading them up with wheat.

On a rotation diet, your child will learn that he can resume enjoying his favorite foods, but with one caveat: He won't be practically living on them as he did in the past. His favorite foods will become *part* of his diet—an occasional part.

As with Step 4 of the elimination diet, the basic purpose of a rotation diet is to test if your child is still sensitive to certain foods. But it is also designed to prevent foods from challenging your child's system and becoming addictive again. If a child resumes eating the same food too frequently, it's more likely that he will develop a reaction to that food. So by rotating foods regularly, you are increasing the variety of foods and combinations of foods that your child is exposed to, which reduces the chance that any old sensitivity will be reactivated or a new one emerge.

Your goal is to replace the onslaught of sensitive foods your child once depended on with healthy choices from other food families that your child likes or needs, and then varying the food within the food family over the course of four days. To test if your child is still sensitive, you will begin with a four-day rotation, in which the offending food is eaten only on the first day of the cycle. You will continue this for four weeks. If there is no reaction as experienced in the past, you will then try a three-day rotation for three weeks, then go to a two-day rotation for two weeks, then down to a one-day rotation for one week. If there is no reaction at all during this time, it means your child's food sensitivity is completely gone and he can go back to eating these foods without repercussions. However, you should still avoid letting the child eat these foods every day. Rotate his diet as best you can.

If at any point during these four-three-two-one-day cycles there is a return of negative symptoms and/or negative behaviors, then you know that one or more foods are still creating a problem. Try to identify the food or foods by rotating them in and out of the diet. If you identify a food, then eliminate it completely from your child's diet for at least six months. Try to reintroduce it again in isolation. If a food continues to produce a negative response, it may be a sign of a genetic weakness and it should be eliminated for good.

We've found that 90 percent of children who come to our Brain Balance Achievement Centers with clear-cut food sensitivities have been able to go back to a completely normal diet after they complete the program and their brain is balanced. We have used this method along with follow-up blood tests to show they are no longer having negative reactions to foods, proving that the source of the food sensitivity was primarily the brain, while the immune system and/or the gut were only secondary players. I like the rotation diet because it guarantees variety and good nutrition and reduces the chance of creating new sensitivities or reactivating old ones. Use plenty of variety at mealtime to ensure that your child is getting vegetables, fruits, and protein-rich foods for optimal nutrition. When considering a rotation diet, make sure each day includes:

- 2 to 4 servings of fruit (a serving is one piece)
- 3 to 5 servings of vegetables (a serving is ½ cup or the equivalent)
- 2 to 4 servings of protein (a serving is 3 to 4 ounces)
- 2 to 3 servings of whole grains (a serving is ½ cup or 1 slice of bread)

Snacks should lean toward fresh fruits, nuts, seeds, and raw veggies.

THERE'S NO REPLACEMENT FOR WATER

Most kids today are walking around chronically dehydrated because they don't get enough water. Water is important for most chemical and metabolic functions, and it helps purify and detoxify the body.

Fruit juice may have water in it, but it is not a substitute for water because it does not react in the body like water. To promote the best for your child's health, offer him or her a full glass of water at every meal.

According to the American Academy of Pediatrics, your child should consume half his weight in ounces of water each day. So a 60-pound child should drink 30 ounces or almost 4 cups of water a day.

BRAIN BALANCE PROFILE
A Change in Bradley's Diet Helped Change Everything

Eight-year-old Bradley walked in to our Brain Balance Achievement Center with his head hung low and his shoulders slumped. He was having trouble reading in school and couldn't understand why. His mother said he would come home from school with blurred vision and headaches—even though the doctor said his eyes were fine—and cry from frustration.

We found that Bradley was quite shy and avoided eye contact. Testing showed he was delayed in all his major motor abilities. He had the gait of a four-year-old. We also found he had a lot of food sensitivities. Gluten, dairy, casein, egg, and mustard were the most severe. In addition to initiating physical exercises, we immediately removed these foods from his diet. That's what made the biggest difference in his life.

Bradley is a great example of why it's important to look for sensitivities and do an elimination diet. Some children have no response at all and others have a huge response—like Bradley. While testing proved he had a brain imbalance and we put him on a motor skills and sensory program, the nutritional aspect seemed to produce the most dramatic changes. Although he still had imbalances in his functions, his headaches and blurred vision improved right away. It was obvious that the foods were playing a very important role in his issues.

Within weeks he was reading without blurred vision and he no longer complained of headaches. Within three months, all his physical delays corrected to his current age level, and in some instances higher.

"Everything, including penmanship, reading, math,

drawing, motor skills, and his sense of smell has improved greatly," his parents later reported. "His self-esteem has improved so much over the last few months and, to us, this in itself is priceless."

The last time we saw Bradley, he was walking with his shoulders back and his head held high!

KNOW YOUR FOOD SUBSTITUTES

Some of the foods kids commonly have sensitivities to are difficult to eliminate because they are found in so many products. This is especially true of dairy, wheat, eggs, and corn. It's also one of the reasons we recommend you avoid packaged and processed foods. If your child has a reaction to any of these foods, you need to be super-diligent about checking ingredient lists. Here's what to look out for:

Dairy
May be listed on labels as:
- Artificial butter flavor
- Butter
- Buttermilk
- Buttermilk solids
- Casein
- Caseinate
- Cheese
- Cottage cheese
- Cream
- Cream cheese
- Half-and-half
- Kefir
- Lactalbumin
- Lactose
- Sodium caseinate
- Sour cream

- Milk
- Milk solids
- Nonfat milk solids
- Whey
- Yogurt

Wheat
May be listed on labels as:
- Bleached flour
- Bulgur
- Cracked wheat
- Durum flour
- Enriched flour
- Farina
- Flour
- Graham flour
- Hard wheat
- Red wheat
- Semolina
- Stone-ground wheat
- Wheat
- Wheat berries
- Wheat bran
- Wheat germ
- Unbleached flour
- Unenriched flour

Eggs
May be listed on labels as:
- Albumin
- Egg protein
- Egg white
- Egg yolk
- Globulin
- Livetin

- Ovomucin
- Ovomucoid
- Ovovitellin
- Ovalbumin
- Powdered egg
- Vitellin

Corn

May be listed on labels as:

- Baking powder
- Glucose syrup
- High-fructose corn syrup
- Hominy
- Maize
- Starch, as in cereal, corn, food, or modified corn starch
- Vegetable, as in vegetable gum, protein, paste, or starch

Soy

May be listed on labels as:

- Hydrolyzed soy protein
- Kinnoko flour
- Kyodofu
- Miso
- Natto
- Okara
- Shoyu albumin
- Soya
- Soybean flour
- Soy butter
- Soy concentrate
- Soy fiber
- Soy grits
- Soy lecithin
- Soy milk
- Soy nuts

- Soy pulp
- Soy sauce
- Soy sprouts
- Supro
- Tamari
- Textured soy flour
- Textured soy protein
- Textured vegetable protein
- Yakidofu
- Yuba

A WORD ABOUT SUGAR

Surprised that sugar is not on our 10 Most Wanted List? Most parents are. Like virtually all parents today and in decades past, they look at "too much sugar" as the source of the tantrums they see played out on a too-regular basis. There is no scientific evidence, though, that sugar is the cause of bad behavior. There is also no evidence that kids can have a sensitivity to sugar as they can to, say, wheat or dairy.

True, too much sugar isn't good for anyone—adults included—and I'll get to that in a moment. But first, I want to tell you the story about sugar and why I allow kids to have it—within reason, of course.

Yes, there has been some research over the years linking intake of sugar with the behavioral issues associated with ADHD. But the results of that research have been mixed. And I have yet to see a child test positive for a sensitivity to sugar, which is why you don't see it on my Most-Wanted List.

You see, it is not sugar itself that is the problem. The issue lies in the way we metabolize sugar—how insulin regulates blood sugar levels. And that's where the brain comes in.

The brain plays a role in sugar metabolism and blood sugar regulation because of the way it drives the stress response. If the brain gets the message that the body is under stress and needs more energy to handle it, it releases cortisol to raise blood glucose. This causes a release of insulin to get the sugar out of the blood stream and into the cells where it can be used for energy. If the brain feels that the body is not in a stressful state, it will reduce blood sugar so the body can calm down, repair itself, and rest.

When a child eats a lot of simple carbohydrates like sugar, blood sugar rises and insulin is released. Cells get so much sugar in them that, initially, the child may become more energetic and even hyperactive, but it is inevitably followed by a crash when blood sugar comes down, causing the child to become cranky and irritable. When this happens too often, it leads to insulin resistance that eventually leads to type 2 diabetes, something we once saw only in older adults but are now starting to see in teens and even young children.

The point I want to make is that sugar isn't the only food that messes with our blood sugar levels. A few years back, T. William Davis, M.D, wrote a fascinating bestselling book called *Wheat Belly*. He highlighted a 1981 University of Toronto study that launched the concept of the glycemic index (GI), which compared foods based on the rate at which they increase the quantity of insulin released and raise blood sugar levels. High GI foods were also related to a higher risk of fat storage. The Index rates foods from 1 through 100, with 50 being in the middle and "moderate." The higher the number, the faster the rate at which blood sugar is released. Interestingly, the GI for white bread is 69; for white table sugar it is only 59. Shredded wheat cereal is 67, and shockingly, whole wheat bread is the worst at 72! In contrast, the GI of a Snickers bar is 41 and a Mars bar, which is the worst of all candy bars, is 68. Therefore wheat products elevate blood sugar more than virtually any other carbohydrate from beans to candy bars. This is why the research on sugar and hyperactivity is so confusing, because sugar doesn't raise blood sugar levels as much as bread does. This is a big revelation!

It means that the thing you need to care about is not sugar, per se, but the effect of blood sugar levels on your child's behavior. Any food that can cause a quick release of blood sugar can lead to hyperglycemia and hyperactivity, followed by a crash of hypoglycemia and irritable behavior.

This is not to say that a child can't have a sensitivity to sugar. A child can have a sensitivity to *any* food. In the case of sugar, however, it is more likely that a brain imbalance is affecting how your child is metabolizing sugar. If you suspect this to be the case, it may be a good idea to avoid or eliminate sugar and only eat foods that are low on the glycemic index until the brain imbalance is corrected. Consider all high-glycemic foods as you would any food sensitivity.

A CAUTION ABOUT ANTIBIOTICS

Candida albicans is a common and usually harmless yeast that lives in the intestinal and urinary tracts. It normally does not produce any difficulty as long as its delicate pH balance is maintained. One thing that can upset the balance is antibiotics.

The problem with antibiotics is that they are so effective that they kill good as well as bad bacteria. In an otherwise healthy child, occasional use of antibiotics is not a problem. However, children with a left-brain imbalance tend to get many infections, especially ear infections, which can expose them to many rounds of antibiotics during their younger years.

Chronic use of antibiotics not only kills the good bacteria necessary for digestion and elimination but also throws off the pH level (acidity) in the intestinal environment that helps suppress the growth of yeast. As a result, yeast can grow unchecked, causing even more infections and symptoms common in FDS. Following are the signs that your child may have a chronic yeast infection:

- Four or more prescriptions for antibiotics within 10 to 12 months
- A prolonged course of antibiotics lasting 4 weeks or longer
- Continuation of symptoms after the infection is cleared
- A craving for sugar
- Persistent digestive problems, including gas, bloating, constipation, or diarrhea

If you suspect your child has a yeast infection, avoid foods that promote the growth of yeast, such as sugar, honey, corn syrup, maple syrup, and brewer's yeast. Avoid yeast-containing foods, which include breads, dried fruit, and cheese.

The best natural way to restore the pH balance in the digestive system is with probiotics, namely *lactobacillus acidophilus*, the culture found in yogurt, and *lactobacillus plantarum*, found in fermented foods. You can also get probiotics in tablet form.

Chapter 4
Feeding Without the Frenzy:
Building a Healthy Relationship with Food

As a parent, some of the most important gifts you can give your child are the tools to healthy eating, but it is a challenge that is compounded significantly when you have a child who is fussy about food.

Out of all the problems our Brain Balance families face—the academic struggles, the family strife, the uncertainties about what the future may hold—my conversations with parents always, and I mean *always*, eventually turn to food. Parents are concerned because their special-needs children refuse to try new foods, will only eat from a very short list of foods, and/or just don't seem to eat enough food. As a result, they worry about their children eating healthily and getting adequate nutrition. How, they often ask, can they get their child to eat a healthy diet?

The answer is: *You have to teach them.*

Parenting by definition involves the responsibility of caring for and feeding one's children. But this has taken on new meaning since earlier times in human evolution, when food scarcity and infectious diseases were the major threats to our children's health. Today, in addition to being faced with an abundance of food, our children are constantly being exposed to a cornucopia of unhealthy junk foods that has largely created a different health threat—childhood obesity and the associated diseases that until recently were never seen in young people, let alone teenagers and adolescents. This has put an unprecedented burden on the shoulders of modern-age parents: protecting their children *from* food in addition to providing them with food. This is why it's more important now than ever that parents act as good food role models. I strongly believe, and there is plenty of research to back me up, that parents are the biggest influence over what their children choose to eat and the dietary habits they will eventually adopt for a lifetime. If you eat healthily and exercise, your children will eat healthily and exercise too. If you are overweight, obese, sedentary, and unhealthy, your child most likely will end up the same way.

"EAT AS I EAT"

Eating healthy food is not something kids come by naturally. You could say it is more of an acquired taste. Scientists have observed this by studying how babies adapt to feeding from infancy through toddlerhood. Shortly after birth, infants are already expressing a preference for the taste of sweet. Fruits, flavored yogurts, and juices are pleasing to them. From the get-go they reject bitter, a flavor component of many vegetables. Laboratory studies have also confirmed that young children readily form a preference for flavors associated with foods higher in calories. For example, the bananas, apples, potatoes, and peas preferred by a lot of kids are fruits and vegetables with a high calorie content.

Biologically, a baby is the same from one culture to the next, but all babies come into this world equipped with a set of behavioral predispositions that allow them to accept the foods made available to them in any particular culture. That's why Chinese toddlers prefer rice and Japanese toddlers prefer udon noodles. We know that part of this influence starts in the womb, where the child can already taste and smell the foods her mother eats, but it's also what children are culturally taught to prefer. It's why so many toddlers in the United States literally cry for French fries and burgers from McDonald's, something you would almost never see in cultures like Greece or Italy. This means that you, the parent, play the leading role in determining what kinds of foods your children will become familiar with and eventually learn to love—from the snacks you keep in your pantry, to the fruits you display on the kitchen counter, to the vegetables you put in your refrigerator, to the meals served at the family table, and especially to the food choices they'll make when away from home.

You also need to act as the gatekeeper over the outside influences that affect your child's eating behavior, from what they are exposed to on television and other media to the habits they could be picking up from their peers at school and play.

The first five years of life are a time of rapid physical growth and change and are the years when eating behaviors are developed that will pave the way to the eating patterns of the future. During these early years, children are learning what, when, and how much to eat based on what they are picking up from the attitudes, habits, and practices they are observing and sensing in their immediate environment—be it the home, the day care center, or the household of whoever is sharing responsibility for your child's upbringing.

There are dozens of ways you can teach your child to have a healthy relationship with food. Here are ways to help you be a better role model, based on what scientific studies have found:

Start Early

A growing body of evidence suggests that the food choices a mother makes during pregnancy may influence an infant's later acceptance of solid foods. Preference for flavor begins very early in life—and therefore so does your food role-modeling. In fact research suggests it may even start in the womb, when a fetus experiences the flavor of the maternal diet during pregnancy and through breast milk during infancy. Amniotic fluid is a rich source of sensory exposure for infants. Because taste and smell are already functional in a fetus, the first experiences with flavor occur prior to birth. For example, one study found detectable odors of garlic, cumin, and curry in the amniotic fluid of pregnant women eating spicy foods.

Promote Family Dinner As an Important Goal

It's 5:30 p.m. and Ben has a baseball game, Olivia's at dance class, and Kennedy is out shopping with friends for a dress for the middle school dance on Friday night. It's another night when everybody will just have to fend for themselves for something to eat.

When your kids are young and they depend on you for their meals, dining together isn't much of an issue, but as kids start to get older and schedules get more hectic, dining together as a family often becomes a challenge. That's why you have to make it a priority. Teenagers actually enjoy dining at home with their parents and siblings, according to The

Importance of Family Dinners VII, a report put out by the National Center on Addiction and Substance Abuse at Columbia University. According to the study, 58 percent of teens report dining as a family five times a week or more, up from 51 percent twelve years ago. What do they enjoy most? Talking, sharing stories, catching up, and spending more time with their parents and siblings.

The center's surveys have consistently found a relationship between frequent family dinners and a decreased risk of children taking up smoking, drinking, and drugs as they get older. According to the report, "parental engagement fostered around the dinner table is one of the most potent tools to help parents raise healthy, drug-free children."

Regular family dinners also foster good mental health in adolescents, according to a study of more than 26,000 kids between the ages of eleven and fifteen. "More frequent family dinners related to fewer emotional and behavioral problems, greater emotional well-being, more trusting and helpful behaviors towards others, and higher life satisfaction," says Frank Elgar, a lead researcher on the study. "We were surprised to find such consistent effects on every outcome we studied. From having no dinners together to eating together seven nights a week, each additional dinner related to significantly better mental health."

This doesn't mean that every family meal will be filled with laughter and mirth. Having family dinner together can be hard and stressful at times, but it is still worth the effort. In the end, it pays off. Always keep in mind that just because it isn't all fun doesn't mean it is not the best thing for your family.

Don't Skip Breakfast Either

An estimated 18 percent of Americans older than age two routinely skip breakfast. This is not a good idea, especially when you consider that breakfast skippers tend to have unhealthy eating habits compared to breakfast eaters. Studies show that young people who skip breakfast consume 40 percent more sweets, 55 percent more soft drinks, 45 percent fewer vegetables, and 30 percent less fruit than young people who eat breakfast.

Limit Meals Away from Home

About 40 percent of family food dollars are now spent on food away from the home. This means your children are being exposed to particularly large portions of calories and fat when dining away from home. One study that examined the dining habits of nearly 10,000 children and adolescents between the ages of 2 and 19 found that they consumed higher amounts of sugar, total fat, saturated fat, and sodium and drank less milk on days they ate at restaurants, adding an extra 309 calories to their daily intake. Other studies found that 41 percent of adolescents and one-third of children between the ages of 2 and 11 consumed fast food on any given day.

Be Authoritative, Not Authoritarian

In other words, don't be a nag. Not only does it not work, it can backfire. Studies reveal that constantly telling your children they need to eat more fruit and vegetables and less junk food has a boomerang effect—they'll end up wanting junk food more often, and when they get the chance to eat it, they'll eat more, even if they aren't hungry. For example, in one study, greater parental pressure was associated with lower intakes of fruits and vegetables and higher intakes of dietary fat, at least among girls. Also, insisting that a child sit at a table until he eats his vegetables most likely will only lead to that child growing up to dislike those vegetables. It's important to maintain a balance, though. Explaining why it is important to eat healthily and making sure that good foods are available to them at each meal will influence their choices. Sometimes, you may have to push them as well.

My wife had a great strategy she used on our kids when they had friends over. Without saying anything she'd put out a plate of cut vegetables and a healthy dipping sauce and just leave it on the table. Before you knew it, it was all gone. It was fun and they enjoyed eating it. It would have been the same if she'd put out chips and dip or French fries. They would have eaten that as well. Often, exposure and presentation make all the difference.

Show by Example

The best way to get your children to eat more vegetables is to set a good example by eating them yourself. If parents load their own plates with colorful vegetables and fruits and leafy greens, the chances are greater that their children will follow suit and do the same, according to several studies conducted by Tanja V.E. Kral Ph.D., of the University of Pennsylvania School of Nursing. "Parents serve as important role models for their children when it comes to healthy eating," says Dr. Kral. "Watching a parent eat initially disliked or novel foods, such as vegetables, can enhance a child's preference for those foods."

Besides modeling healthy eating behaviors, as a parent it is up to you to decide what foods to make available to your children at home. Making vegetables easily accessible offers your kid the opportunity to try new foods and to taste them repeatedly. "It is important to know that children's innate taste preferences can be modified through repeated experiences with food," says Dr. Kral. "Studies have shown that multiple exposures to the taste of initially disliked or novel foods can significantly increase children's liking and acceptance of those foods, including vegetables."

If You Don't Want Them to Eat It, Don't Keep It in the House

Kids should not have open access to any snack or food they want at any time they want. I see this way too often. Too many kids today have unregulated access to high-calorie, low-nutrition snacks, which undoubtedly is contributing to our childhood obesity epidemic. It's the same with screen time. Both need to be regulated and controlled by the parent. I recommend two simple rules:

- If there are foods you do not want your kids to eat, do not keep them in the house.
- Establish a system whereby your child must ask permission to eat a snack.

Be firm and stick to your goals. In many ways, good parenting is being willing to fight, to be uncomfortable, and to not take the easy way out. This is especially important with food choices and meals. Being successful at anything is about being comfortable with being uncomfortable. Being a good parent is about being comfortable with your children being uncomfortable. Many parents today can't stand to see their children struggle, so they immediately try to fix things, and that's unfortunate. They don't want to fight with their children to eat their veggies or to not eat junk food, so they let their kids eat what they want. And that's unfortunate too. This kind of attitude is hurting kids more than it helps. As a result, many kids today don't have self-control or coping skills because we never let them struggle and figure things out for themselves.

Don't give in if your child rejects a new food. If your child has a sensory processing disorder, getting her to try a new food can take quite a bit of effort, and I offered a solution on page 34 that we've found works. With other children, however, it is just a matter of patience on your part. The tendency for children to reject a new food is often just a case of *neophobia*, the fear of something new. Several studies have found that a child's preference for and acceptance of a new food is enhanced with repeated exposure to the food in a nonauthoritarian setting. In preschool-age children, it can take from ten to sixteen exposures before you witness acceptance. Most parents give up after only two or three tries.

BRAIN BALANCE PROFILE
The Foods Amelia Loved Didn't Love Her Back

Amelia seemed like a normal, happy, and healthy baby, but around the age of eighteen months her mother noticed she wasn't hitting some of the milestones of other children her age. She was doing well in some other areas, so her mother brushed them aside. For one thing, Amelia was a great eater, then suddenly started to get very picky. Soon all she would eat was toast, cheese, milk, and eggs. Sometimes she would only calm down by drinking her sippy cup of milk sitting behind a certain chair in the corner of the room.

When Amelia was twenty months old, her grandmother declared her a wunderkind because she could name all the letters, colors, and shapes. By age two she was doing one hundred–piece puzzles and memory games with little assistance, but she struggled in other areas of life. She was so obsessed with princesses that her parents decided to take her to Disneyland where, to their surprise, she wouldn't go near them. It was almost as if they frightened her. "When we took her on one ride she absolutely could not handle it and was screaming and clawing at me to get out," her mother said. "It was very clear that something was not right."

Her parents were told Amelia had Asperger's syndrome. They were devastated. They took her from doctor to doctor and got one evaluation after another. They experimented with diets and saw some improvements, but still the odd behaviors persisted. Eventually she showed up at one of our Brain Balance Achievement Centers.

When we first met Amelia we could see that she had retreated into her own world and showed very little emotion. She was socially awkward. Testing showed she had a severe right-brain imbalance. We also found she had a lot of food sensitivities, including wheat, dairy, and eggs—the very foods she craved. We started her on an elimination diet along with the multimodal Brain Balance Program, and within weeks her mother noticed marked improvement.

After completing the program, her mother wrote: "Our little girl began to open up and take notice of others! Her behaviors improved, she responded to discipline the way other children her age do, and she began to finally enjoy new foods. Amelia is now in school, and every day she runs to her classroom waving and giggling with friends. She is once again a happy, healthy little girl."

SPOTLIGHT ON BEHAVIOR

The most common mistake parents make at mealtime is to feed Mom and Dad one thing—let's say pork chops, peas, and potatoes—and their kids something else—let's say pasta (what else!). This is the worst thing you can do. Giving in to your kid's demands for a different meal creates a problem, because the child now understands this as, *If I complain, Mommy or Daddy will then feed me what I want.* This is not the type of message you want to send. Rather, you should start out by getting the message across that *Mom and Dad are not short-order cooks.* Your children should understand that they are not permitted to swap out a healthy dinner for a hot dog, pasta, pizza, or any other food of *their* choice. Once that is established, here's how you can go about establishing more discipline at mealtime:

Make Meals Child-Friendly

Pleasant mealtimes work out better when you start off with a food that you know your child will eat willingly. For example, expecting a child, especially a fussy child, to eat lamb is a bit of a stretch. Chicken is a much safer bet. This way, you are not setting yourself up for failure. Your child will feel good about herself for being able to meet her goals, and you will feel good about praising her in a positive way.

Reward, Reward, Reward, but Never with or About Food

I am a big fan of a reward system, especially where it involves behavior. I tell parents to "catch your child being good" and reward the behavior. I like the idea of using stickers. For example, sitting through a meal without fidgeting or getting up without permission can mean a gold star in your child's sticker book or on the family bulletin board. However, never use dessert, a before-bed treat, or any unhealthy or calorie-dense food as a lure. Studies show that using sweet, palatable foods as rewards can have the unintended consequence of promoting a child's preference for unhealthy high-calorie foods.

By the same token, don't consider that eating a healthy meal is deserving of a reward in itself. Rather, consider that it's what's to be expected—*it's normal*. Rewarding children for eating a healthy meal in the hope that it will interest them in eating more vegetables can actually backfire. One study found this practice resulted in children learning to dislike vegetables.

Don't Put Restrictions on Certain "Junk" Foods as a Means to Promote Healthy Eating

If you don't want your child to eat certain foods, then don't keep them in the house—ever. Keeping "restricted" food in the house but out of reach can also produce unintended results. Studies show that edicts such as *you may have just one cookie* or *you can have just one small handful of chips* decreases a child's ability to practice restraint when she is permitted around the food—even if she isn't hungry. One study involving middle-class white families with daughters ages five through nine found that restrictive family practices such as this resulted in "uninhibited overeating and greater weight gain."

Eat at the Same Time Every Day

It helps if you make an effort to eat at the same time each day. When children eat in a timely manner, they become more comfortable with their routine. This is important for children with sensory issues as well as kids who are fussy around food. In addition, they will begin to be hungry at these times, since their bodies respond to such a schedule by producing digestive enzymes around the time they are used to eating.

Ignore Inappropriate Behaviors

If your child is acting badly at the table, no matter how annoying it is, try to ignore it. Counteract it by rewarding good behaviors. Here's an example of how this can work:

Brian has a plate of mashed potatoes and peas set before him. His mother, Penny, has a tough time getting him to eat the peas, and Brian finally decides to throw them. Mom continues to try to force the peas and finally Brian throws a tantrum. Brian only wants to eat the potatoes.

You can't just ignore this kind of behavior, and it should be reprimanded. However, let's say Penny decides to try a different approach.

First, she feeds Brian the mashed potatoes that she knows he'll eat and praises him by giving him a hug. Brian takes more potatoes and is happy. Then Mom decides to try again for the peas. Surprisingly, Brian tries them. Mom is very happy and praises Brian again.

The above example is fantastic when everything goes well. Sometimes, the opposite happens and things don't go very well.

If your child is spitting food out at you, try turning his chair around for a few minutes facing the wall. This will give him the idea that you will not pay attention to him while he is behaving this way. Turn the chair back around and offer the food again. If he eats it, great. You are on the correct track. Give it another try and if it doesn't work, send the child to his room without eating. Eventually he will learn that he is to eat what is made for him or he will go hungry.

The important point here is that if the child tries, you should reward the effort with lots of positive feedback and praise. As with almost everything, it is most important to reward the effort, not the result. This teaches kids that the most important thing is to try and to not be afraid to try new things. Consistency is key, and eventually, virtually all children will master this concept.

Use Positive Reinforcements

Positive reinforcement can be a very effective tool. For example:

- Tell your children to pick out a game and tell them they can play it after dinner if *all* of them behave as expected during dinner.
- Have your child tie on an apron and pitch in to prepare dinner. Most times, children will get excited about a meal they help prepare.
- Make up a contract stating that you expect your child to eat specific portions of food at each meal—for example, a whole sandwich, a piece of fruit, carrot sticks, and so forth. For each week that she eats correctly, offer a reward— a trip to the movies or a special toy.

PUTTING SENSORY SENSITIVITIES IN THE MIX

Granted, promoting healthy eating and instituting family dinners, especially what you envision to be normal gatherings, can be tough when you have a problem feeder in the mix. It is even more challenging to teach healthy eating habits to an entire family when you are worried about one child who doesn't want to eat at all. In addition to the suggestions for specific sensory issues offered in Chapter 2, we have found that you can help a child feel more comfortable with food by making it look and seem like fun. Here are some methods we use at Brain Balance and recommend that parents employ at home.

Become More Hands-On with Foods

Show your child how fun it can be to squish food, stir it, smell it, pour it into different containers, and dump it out again. Pour applesauce or yogurt on a large cutting board or kitchen counter (if you don't mind the mess) and let your child finger paint with it or just make a big mess. Any type of interaction you can get is great. Getting hands-on allows your child to see that food is fun and safe to touch and eat.

If your child has trouble having direct contact with foods, you can always cover his hands in latex gloves or plastic wrap. Or try getting him closer to it by using paintbrushes to explore the food. Paint with pudding, applesauce, baby food, condiments, or any other spreadable food.

Create Food Art

Encourage your child to create a picture of a person or an animal with food. For example, use M&Ms for eyes, jelly beans to make a nose, pretzel sticks to form eyebrows, and licorice strings to make a mouth.

Explore a Little

Pique your child's interest in foods by getting her interested in textures and tastes. Create a food chart categorizing foods into textures, shapes, and colors, such as crunchy, soft, smooth, slimy, tough, rough, bumpy, tart, squishy, tart, and sweet.

Put a Toy Kitchen in Your Home Kitchen

Involve your child in the whole food experience by getting a toy kitchen that you can place in your kitchen and have your child follow along and mimic you while you prepare a meal.

Get Your Child More Involved Creatively

Start by taking your child along to go food shopping. If you really want to get creative, have your child paste pictures of what you're going to buy from the store circular in your local newspaper onto your grocery list. Have her find the item for you in the produce section and check it off the list. Praise her for a job well done.

Start a Kid's Vegetable Garden

Starting a kid's vegetable garden is a great way to get your finicky child interested in eating vegetables. Help him plant, water, and cultivate his very own veggie garden. You will find most children are very excited to get involved in this process and are willing to try eating something they've grown themselves.

Innovate Playtime Around Food

Any games you can play involving food will help your child feel more comfortable around food. Have your child host a tea party for friends. Play restaurant before dinner, allowing your child to take orders from family members. Play Kid's Deli using toy sandwiches and a toy cash register. Buy some coloring and connect-the-dot books that focus on food.

Cook with Your Child

Learning to cook is such a great milestone for a child. Most children are very excited to eat whatever they have prepared. My wife always encouraged our kids to cook. They now love to cook healthy but very tasty foods, especially spicy foods. When they were young, helping Mom cook was a great outlet for their energy, helping them concentrate and be creative at the same time. They now feel totally comfortable in the kitchen, and this helps them to be independent and autonomous.

THE PARENTAL CODE FOR KEEPING YOUR COOL

There is always a way to find calm amidst chaos if you take the extra measure to enforce discipline around mealtime. But here I mean *self*-discipline.

When things seems to get out of hand, take a deep breath and restrain yourself from yelling. Gather your composure and remember to:

Be consistent. If you are not consistent, your child will not be. Once a set of rules is enforced, be sure to stick to it. It can be helpful to keep a written chart of all of the things you expect from your child on a white board or bulletin board so that they are visible and not "forgotten."

Make a vow to say things only once. No parent wants to constantly repeat himself. Kneel down to your child's level and look him in the eye when you are explaining things or reprimanding him.

Believe you can do it, and commit to the effort. This is sometimes referred to as The Law of Attraction— namely, that you can achieve anything if you firmly believe in it and take the actions necessary to make it happen. Waffling, compromising, and giving up are not an option when you commit to staying the course. The results will surprise you.

ACCEPTING NEW FOODS: A NEW "CHAIN" OF EVENTS

Let's now get back to that vexing, perplexing problem that's most likely at the source of much of the family strife you are experiencing at mealtime: a child with a very limited interest in food. We have found that it *is* possible to get a fussy eater and even a problem feeder to try and even like new foods. The process is called *food chaining* and is based on a book by the same name created by four specialists to help stop picky eating and ease mealtime dilemmas. We modified the process to meet the needs of children with brain imbalances and sensory discrimination disorders. We like it because we've found it to be a highly effective way to get children to accept new foods in a gradual and nonthreatening way. It is a process you can undertake after your child has completed the elimination and rotation diet.

Food chaining is actually a fairly simple process. It is based on the idea that your child will eat only what he likes. This is true of everyone, but for some kids, the list is simply too short and not acceptable. A food chain works because it introduces new foods into the diet by gradually building on the flavors and textures your child already prefers.

Review Your Child's Diet

Look at the foods your child consistently eats at home, school, and/or at day care. This is what we call his *core diet*. What you want to identify are patterns in taste, texture, temperature, and consistency that constitute his core diet. Generally, the foods your child eats day in and day out all possess some commonality. Perhaps the foods he loves tend to be either sweet, spicy, crunchy, or salty. For example, he may like cereal that is crunchy and dry and hate cereal that is soft, creamy, and wet like oatmeal. What patterns do you notice in the foods your child likes?

My child's food preference tends to lean more toward:

- ☐ Sweet
- ☐ Hot/spicy
- ☐ Crunchy
- ☐ Salty
- ☐ Bland
- ☐ Pungent
- ☐ A combination of several of the above

Next, think back to some of the foods your child ate in the past and now rejects. Knowing what you now know about your child's taste preference, what is it telling you? If your child once liked pancakes and doesn't anymore, but also likes crunchy foods, maybe you can transition her to French toast or waffles. To transition from one new food to the next, you want to look for foods that are as close as possible in taste, texture, shape, et cetera to foods your child is already comfortable with.

To start, make a list of the foods your child currently accepts:

_____

_____

_____

_____

_____

_____

For the purposes of this exercise, let's use this list as an example:

- Chicken fingers
- Macaroni and cheese
- Cola
- Apple juice
- Potato chips
- French fries
- Milk

Starting the Food Chain

Select a food from the list. To make this procedure less overwhelming to the senses, you will want to work on this by changing only one food at a time. Altering more than one food at a time can be quite overwhelming for a child and cause her to become scared and regress.

Get your child involved in the process by explaining what you are going to do. It will be much easier for your child to transition if you begin speaking to her about her new food evolution a week or so before introducing a new type of food or food group. You can start off by describing how the food tastes or smells.

For our example, I've chosen the chicken fingers. At the first meal, feed her the chicken fingers the way she likes them. Let's assume this is a packaged brand you purchase frozen at the supermarket. At the following meal in which you'd serve chicken fingers, transition to a better-quality brand, preferably one that is organic and/or free of pesticides. This serves two purposes: Your child is still enjoying her favorite food and texture but the quality of the food is improving. She may balk a bit (or more) about the change, but continue to serve them until she is comfortable with them. Be patient, as it could take a while. Next, try another brand and go through the same process. Finally, go to a homemade variety, such as the Coconut-Crusted Chicken Fingers recipe we feature on page 145.

No matter what type of food you choose to work with, always end up with a homemade dish, something in which you are in control of the ingredients and the nutrients. "Hiding" nutrition in homemade dishes is a fabulous idea for fussy eaters and a great way to develop growing taste buds. Such a concept was introduced in Jessica Seinfeld's bestselling book *Deceptively Delicious* and Missy Lapine's *The Sneaky Chef.* These books present the ingenious idea of disguising vegetables in common children's foods. For example, when preparing chicken nuggets, instead of using egg to dredge the chicken (which most children with a brain imbalance can't tolerate anyway), use organic baby spinach puree. No one would ever know the difference, and you end up giving your child the gift of additional vitamins and minerals they normally would not get.

Once the child has become accustomed to your "new" chicken fingers, you can start experimenting more. Small changes, like less breading or more breading, will vary the texture from crunchy to soft. You can also add different herbs or rice cheese to the breadcrumbs to come up with a more flavorful taste. Once your child accepts this, you can move onto chicken breasts instead of fingers.

Next, move on to different proteins. Instead of chicken, try fish. Fish is an excellent source of protein, and many varieties contain high levels of brain-supporting omega-3 fatty acids. From protein, you'll be ready to kick it up another notch: Bring on the vegetables! Zucchini, eggplant, squash, and onions all take well to breading.

Keep in mind that if your goal is to get your child to eat meat, this could be a difficult process. Many children have a hard time chewing and breaking down meats like roast beef, pot roast, venison, and pork. Sometimes even lunch meat can be hard for a child to eat. If you notice your child is having difficulty, you can opt for softer proteins like chicken, turkey, and fish. You can also try pureeing meats and gradually transitioning to a denser consistency.

You can also try to add condiments along with the new variety of breaded fare, such as organic ketchup, mustard, chili sauce, tartar sauce, various dressings, vinaigrettes, and sauces. Try Stacey's All-Natural Homemade Ketchup on page 143.

The next step in the process is the big one. You're going to abandon the breading and serve a simple chicken tender with the ketchup. Coupling the now-familiar ketchup with the slightly unfamiliar chicken without breading is another giant step leading to a big transition.

If at first you don't succeed, try, try again. This can be the best way to reposition a new food so your child will now accept it. If all else fails, consider hiding the food. For example, if your child loves macaroni and cheese, add some butternut squash to it. The color and texture are almost completely the same, so mostly likely your child will not notice. You can also try mixing spaghetti squash in with regular pasta and adding sauce to cover. It is very possible your child will be none the wiser!

If you have a child with a severe sensory issue, this process can take some time. For some children it might have to begin with working up a tolerance to just being in the same room with a certain food. As already noted in Chapter 2, you may have to start off with your child merely accepting touching a food or putting it to his lips. Even if the child just licks the food and does not eat it, this can be considered progress.

Just remember, slow and steady wins the race.

YOUR HEALTHY SHOPPING STRATEGY

To make your family meals healthier, follow these food-shopping guidelines. You can't go wrong:

- Spend the most time in the produce section, the first and largest area you encounter in most supermarkets. Choose a rainbow of colorful fruits and vegetables to reflect a variety of vitamin, mineral, and phytonutrient content.
- Go organic on everything. Though it costs more, avoiding pesticides is imperative when dealing with a child with a compromised immune system, an underdeveloped gut, and the other issues that are part of having a brain imbalance.
- Choose grains that are the least processed—for example, regular oatmeal rather than instant—and steer clear of anything containing gluten. Buy whole grains containing at least 4 grams of fiber per serving. The less sugar, the better.
- Go for nondairy calcium-fortified alternatives to milk, such as rice, coconut, almond, or other nut milks.
- When it comes to meat, fish, and poultry, the American Heart Association recommends two servings of fish a week. Buy only wild-caught fish, as farm-raised fish have higher levels of toxins that can affect the brain. Salmon is a great choice because it is not too fishy and is a good source of omega-3 fatty acids. Choose lean cuts of meat (like round, top sirloin, and tenderloin), and opt for skinless poultry. Think small portions when buying and serving.
- Remember that frozen fruits and vegetables without sauce are a convenient way to help fill in the produce gap, especially in winter.

- When cruising the center aisles, where the canned and packaged foods reside, look for foods with as little processing and as few additives as possible. For example, choose only 100 percent fruit juice and 100 percent whole grains. As a rule of thumb, avoid foods containing more than five ingredients, artificial ingredients, or ingredients you can't pronounce. Steer clear of foods with cartoons on the label that are targeted to children. If you don't want your kids eating junk foods, don't have them in the house.
- Keep a variety of canned vegetables, fruits, and beans on hand to toss into soups, salads, whole grain pastas, and rice dishes. Whenever possible, choose vegetables without added salts and fruit packed in natural juice.
- Tuna packed in water, low-fat soups, nut butters, olive and canola oils, and assorted vinegars should be in every healthy pantry.

Chapter 5
Fueling Your Child with Brain Nutrition

Children's diets are notoriously bad, but as the parent of a child who is developmentally challenged, you already know this—in spades. What you may not fully realize, however, is that poor nutrition is a major threat to the developing brain.

Your child's brain can get all the proper stimulation it needs to grow, but it won't be able to make good use of it without the right amount of fuel it needs. Without fuel, too much stimulation can actually end up damaging or killing brain cells. Without stimulation, the body cannot properly break down food and absorb the necessary nutrients needed as fuel. The two must work synergistically. You can follow the Brain Balance exercises you learned about in *Disconnected Kids* to a tee, but your child's true potential will not be realized unless you follow through on the nutritional part of the program. That's why this book, and this chapter in particular, are so important.

That said, here's the reassuringly good news: There is nothing special about the kinds of foods that are healthy for the brain. They are the exact same foods *all* children need for optimum overall health—body *and* brain. The most important foods for a child with the disorders discussed in this book are a variety of vegetables, fruits, nuts, and seeds to improve microbiota diversity and support gut immune tolerance. This means avoiding gluten and dairy and limiting simple and processed sugars. It also means focusing on the nutrients that improve brain performance.

WHAT THE BRAIN NEEDS
Nutrition for adequate development of the brain and body requires a mix of forty-five nutritional elements, including vitamins, minerals, amino acids, essential fatty acids, water, and complex carbohydrates. Studies are coming

out almost weekly showing that children with neurological disorders, particularly ADHD and autism, have deficiencies in amino acids, essential fatty acids, and a variety of vitamins and minerals. Sure, studies reveal that the majority of *all* kids today eat too many simple carbohydrates in the form of junk food and are sorely missing out on the complex carbohydrates found in whole grains. But studies are also revealing that children with the neurological disorders that come under the umbrella of FDS fare much worse than typical children. This may not be due only to poor dietary choices but also to the nutritional malabsorption caused by a leaky gut. For example:

- Studies show that antioxidant stores are low in children with autism, suggesting that these children may be compromised in their ability to metabolize the nutrients, which may be further handicapped by a faster rate of oxidative stress.
- A study published in the journal *Pediatrics* that followed the parent-reported dietary habits of children with autism found they had below the daily recommended intake of nine essential vitamins and minerals, including brain-building vitamins A and D and the minerals calcium, magnesium, and potassium.
- A study of 191 elementary school children, reported in the Journal *Nutrients,* found "a significant association" between a traditional healthy diet—that is, low in fat and high in complex carbohydrates as well as fatty acids and minerals—and lower odds of having ADHD.
- One study that compared 100 children with ADHD to 100 children with healthy brain function found that those with the brain imbalance were "significantly lower" in these brain-healthy nutrients: calcium, iron, magnesium, selenium, zinc, vitamin B-6, folate, niacin, and thiamine.
- An Asian study that examined the dietary habits of 417 students with ADHD found that those who ate a diet high in processed meat and salty snacks scored high on an index of hyperactive behavior. Those who ate healthier foods, such as vegetables, whole-grain cereals, and fish had lower scores.

- A study on children taking the generic form of Ritalin for ADHD found that their daily calorie and nutritive intake was significantly lower than in the general same-age population. They were ingesting less protein, carbohydrates, fats, fiber, calcium, iron, magnesium, zinc, selenium, and B vitamins.
- A review of fifty-two studies that examined dietary changes for the reduction of symptoms in ADHD found that an elimination diet and fish oil supplementation "seem to be the most promising dietary intervention for the reduction in ADHD symptoms in children."
- A study on children and adolescents in developed countries found that they perform better on tests of nonverbal intelligence and on behavioral measures after receiving vitamin and mineral supplements for three months, regardless of age and the formula. The strongest effects were seen in children with ADHD and learning disabilities.
- A study of 20 children with autism conducted by the Autism Research Institute found that more than 50 percent had low levels of
  - vitamins A, B-1, B-3, B-5, and biotin
  - minerals selenium, zinc, and magnesium
  - essential fatty acids
  - two fatty acids, omega-3 and omega-6

Virtually all of these problems manifest themselves because children with these neurological condition do not absorb nutrients well, even if they are eating a perfect diet! To offset these unique challenges facing parents of children with FDS, we recommend a complete nutritional plan as part of the Brain Balance multimodal program. It includes a healthy eating plan and supplement program based on the nutrients that support and promote healthy brain development. These same foods will also nurture the brain throughout life, which is why you can and should consider this a family approach. They are all common everyday foods—the same foods you find in any healthy diet. In fact, the brains of *all* children would benefit from eating this way.

Our Brain Balance Achievement Centers are learning centers, and we do not put a lot of emphasis on diet and food. In my personal practice, however, I do counsel parents about supplements because, as I pointed out earlier, the nature of a leaky gut leaves children nutritionally deficient. The types of supplements a child may need are very individual and can only be ascertained after taking a detailed history and doing lab work. If you feel your child needs supplemental nutritional help, I recommend you see a specialist in functional neurology or functional nutrition to design a program, as the typical physician is not trained in nutrition or well versed in nutritional knowledge, and most experts in autism and other neurodevelopmental disorders are not nutrition experts and may not understand the interrelationship between these conditions and a leaky gut.

This chapter is meant to be informative only. *It is not prescriptive.* It is designed to showcase the nutrients that are essential to brain health and give you all the necessary background on them should you find your child needs supplemental assistance. For most nutrients, you will notice the dosages I recommend vary greatly in range. This is because the exact amount—*to be determined only by an expert*—is determined by the size of the child and the severity of the deficiency.

Keep in mind that a poor diet is a well-researched trigger for exacerbating many of the symptoms associated with most of the conditions that come under the umbrella of FDS. If you find it necessary to supplement, it should only be done for the short term, or until the brain is balanced and functioning at a proper level. As your child's digestive system develops and she sheds her food sensitivities, absorption of these much-needed nutrients will improve until supplements are no longer necessary. You will be able to detect this through the improvement you see in your child's behavior, social skills, and learning ability and achievements—all signs that the brain is getting in sync. If your child is functioning in school, at home, and on the playground at an age-appropriate level, then she probably doesn't need to take high doses of vitamins or specialized supplements. A good multivitamin and a healthy diet should suffice. Food is always more important than supplements! While you will eventually be able to reintroduce many and most likely all of the foods your child is currently sensitive to, you will want to continue focusing your meals on the other foods we've identified as promoting brain health. This doesn't mean your child must eat *only* these foods; it means you should strive to feed your child as many of them as possible as part of a well-balanced diet throughout the day. A healthy diet containing a variety of natural foods is best.

BRAIN BALANCE PROFILER
Gabriel Smells Cookies for the First Time

Gabriel was six when his mother brought him to see me. I was impressed with her right away. She was extremely knowledgeable and had committed all of her time and resources to finding ways to help her son, who had been diagnosed with both moderate autism and ADHD.

When I first evaluated Gabriel, he had severe language difficulties. He didn't communicate much and would repetitively say phrases he had heard on the television. It was clear, however, that he had no real understanding of the words he was constantly repeating.

Gabriel would not make eye contact with me. His mother told me that he was this way with everybody. If I turned my back just for a second, he would make a run for it. I was often chasing him down the hall to bring him back to our sessions. He also had no sense of smell and a fast heart rate for his age, which was very puzzling to his pediatrician. He was physically stressed out.

Gabriel unquestionably had the classic signs of autism. I started to work with him by doing a number of physical exercises and sensory-stimulation exercises directed at activating his right brain.

Testing also revealed that Gabriel had moderate to severe sensitivities to a number of foods, most notably dairy, wheat, and eggs. So we took him off these foods and changed his diet in other ways to make it more nutritious.

Six weeks into the Brain Balance Program, his mother brought him to a session with tears of joy. "I just had my first real conversation with my son," she said. From that time on, Gabriel showed significant positive changes in his behavior, motor, and academic skills. He also started to develop a sense of smell. His mom was thrilled to report, "For the first time I saw him inhale the aroma of freshly baked chocolate-chip cookies."

At the end of twelve weeks, his mother brought me his report card. Earlier in the school year and prior to coming to Brain Balance he was getting all Rs, for Requires Support. Now he had all Ms, for Meets Expectations. She was ecstatic.

At about this time we also redid blood tests to check his food sensitivities. His wheat sensitivity had gone away, and he now showed only a slight sensitivity to dairy. This was a sign that his digestive system was functioning better and his immune system was not as hyperactive. His pediatrician reported that his heart rate was now normal.

NUTRITION FOR THE BRAIN

These are the nutrients that help promote brain development and health and the kid-friendly foods that are high in such nutrients. I want to make one thing clear, though: For most of these nutrients, other foods exist that may contain greater amounts, but they didn't make these lists because they are either on the food-sensitivity list you read about in Chapter 3 or because they get a nearly universal thumbs-down as a food kids will like or even be willing to try.

VITAMIN A BRAIN BENEFITS

Vitamin A, a powerful antioxidant most recognized for eye health, is even more important to the brain. It is essential throughout life for proper brain function. Specifically, it is a potent signaling molecule for brain development; helps regulate the production of various genes, including those involved in brain building; is instrumental in the processes resulting in neuron production; and is involved in the communication network in the brain. One study, reported in the *Journal of the American Dietetic Association*, found that vitamin A was among the nutrients least likely to be consumed in adequate amounts among children on the autism spectrum.

Recommended Amount

10,000 IU (international units). Vitamin A is a fat-soluble vitamin, meaning it is absorbed by, rather than excreted from, the body and can be toxic at high levels. To get this amount of vitamin A without concerns for toxicity, you can supplement with 10 milligrams of beta-carotene, a form of vitamin A.

Top Kid-Friendly Vitamin A Foods

Vitamin A is abundant in many foods. It is highest in liver and oily fish, although these are not on any kid-friendly lists we've ever seen. It is also found in milk and eggs, which will not be available to your child during the elimination diet and possibly even longer if one or both turn out to be a problem food. All leafy greens also contain plenty of vitamin A. In fact, when looking for vitamin A, look for the colors orange, red, and dark green—a sign of vitamin A and pro-vitamin A, the well-known antioxidant beta-carotene. These are the foods we like for their vitamin A content:

- Broccoli
- Cantaloupe
- Carrots
- Dried apricots
- Liver
- Mango
- Pumpkin (see recipe for Pumpkin Pie Muffins on page 130)
- Red bell peppers
- Spinach
- Sweet potatoes

ABOUT DOSAGES

The dosages of nutrients recommended in my books and in my practice are greater than what you see recommended by the federal government and on nutritional labels as the Daily Value (DV) or Recommended Dietary Allowance (RDA).

One reason is that the DV or RDA is considered to be the *minimum* needed to prevent a deficiency, not what is best for optimum health. Optimal recommended dosages can vary, and there is a litany of arguments both for and against mega-dosing.

In my practice, we look at vitamins, minerals, and other nutrients from the perspective of brain health. Because of the digestive difficulties inherent in children with brain imbalances, getting the optimal nutrition for brain health is extremely important. Simply put, much of the nutrition a child gets from food is not being absorbed properly and getting to the brain where it is needed. This is why you will see dosages recommended that are much higher than the DV or RDA.

VITAMIN B-12 BRAIN BENEFITS

Vitamin B-12 is essential for the growth and stability of neurons. It is involved in the production of nerve cells and for manufacturing the myelin sheaths that protect the nerves. It also helps reduce levels of the toxic amino acid homocysteine. High levels of homocysteine are an indicator of faulty methylation, a critical process in the brain that helps maintain the right chemical balance. High levels of homocysteine are common in many children with FDS, especially those who have been diagnosed with autism. A B-12 deficiency can interfere with the brain's ability to produce protective myelin sheaths. Short-term deficiency can cause fatigue and lethargy, but long-term deficiency can result in damage to the brain and central nervous system. Stores of vitamin B-12 can be low in children who are not getting any dairy, cheese, or eggs in their diet, as these foods are a major source of the vitamin. Studies also show low B-12 status in children with autism. And several studies have found B-12 to be deficient in children who do not take supplements.

Recommended Amount
100 to 1,000 mcgs.

Top Kid-Friendly Vitamin B-12 Foods
There are no vegetable sources of natural vitamin B-12, so if your problem feeder has an aversion to them, you'd think offering some other way to get this common nutrient would be a breeze. Unfortunately, some of the richest sources of B-12 are also "sensitivity foods"—mainly the aforementioned milk, cheese, and eggs. Then there's the fact that some of the biggest B-12 boosters are foods that are an acquired taste for most kids: liver, mackerel, and mollusks. Announce you're having mackerel for dinner and see how fast the room clears! There are plenty of ways to get an ample supply of B-12 in your family's diet, however, as it is readily available in all "flesh foods" and in fortified cereals. Try these foods:

- Beef, especially chuck
- Chicken
- Fortified cereals
- Salmon
- Shellfish, especially clams and crabs
- Tuna
- Turkey
- Veal

VITAMIN B-6 BRAIN BENEFITS
Also known as pyridoxine, B-6 is essential to the production of neurotransmitters, the chemicals that allow the brain and nerve cells to communicate with one another. It is also necessary for the proper functioning

of key metabolic processes, and acts as a coenzyme in the breakdown and utilization of carbohydrates, fat, and protein. Along with vitamin B-12, it helps reduce homocysteine levels.

Though controversial, large doses of vitamin B-6 both alone and in conjunction with magnesium have been found to reduce symptoms of autism and pervasive developmental disorder (PDD). Studies appear to establish that supplemental vitamin B-6 can benefit as many as half of children with autism, and safety and efficacy are improved when it is combined with magnesium.

Recommended Amount
20 to 60 mgs.

Top Kid-Friendly Vitamin B-6 Foods
Many of the foods that are the richest in vitamin B-6 happen to be the foods you find most often on the dinner table. They include:

- Banana
- Beef
- Chicken
- Pistachios
- Salmon
- Spinach
- Sunflower seeds
- Sweet potatoes
- Tuna
- Turkey

THIAMINE (VITAMIN B-1) BRAIN BENEFITS
Thiamine is important to every tissue in the body, but it has its biggest impact on two vital organs—the brain and the heart. It is indispensible for making neurotransmitters and for normal nerve function. It is a chief source of energy production, so it helps keep the brain sharp. It's known as the "antistress vitamin" because of its ability to boost the immune system. Thiamine is an important nutrient for kids with FDS because it aids in improving

---

"B" IS FOR BRAIN

Think of the B-vitamin family as brain food. All the B vitamins play a crucial role in brain function, from manufacturing neurotransmitters to regulating energy release in brain cells. All the Bs are necessary to convert the food we eat to glucose, the brain's chief source of fuel. Deficiencies of vitamins B-6, B-12, and folic acid in particular have been found in children diagnosed with autism. Strive to get a variety of foods high in B vitamins in your kid's meals each day.

---

digestive problems and helps increase appetite in those who aren't interested in eating. Anecdotally, it is believed to promote a positive attitude.

Recommended Amount
50 to 100 mgs.

Top Kid-Friendly Thiamine Foods
Thiamine is found in a variety of both plant and animal foods, though unfortunately we mostly get it through eating wheat-based breads and pastas, beans and other legumes, and milk, which are all on the sensitivity list. Rather, the top foods to reach for to get thiamine are:

- Almonds and macadamia nuts
- Asparagus
- Beef
- Pork
- Rice and rice bran
- Salmon
- Sunflower seeds
- Tuna
- Winter squash

NIACIN (VITAMIN B-3) BRAIN BENEFITS

Niacin is important to overall health and the healthy maintenance of brain cells. Studies show it helps in the synthesis and repair of DNA, plays a role in signaling between nerve cells, and acts as a potent antioxidant in brain cells. Niacin seems to have a particularly potent role in maintaining mental agility and appears to have a calming effect on children.

Recommended Amount

10 to 50 mgs, taken in the supplemental form niacinimide.

Top Kid-Friendly Niacin Foods

Niacin is found in a variety of foods, especially meats. Other rich sources are dairy, eggs, wheat, and legumes, which can make getting enough niacin through food alone particularly challenging. Instead, look to these foods as a source of niacin:

- Asparagus
- Avocado
- Bacon (noncured, organic, and chemical free)
- Bell peppers
- Broccoli
- Chicken breast
- Portobello mushroom
- Rice bran
- Sweet potatoes
- Tuna (yellow fin)

PANTOTHENIC ACID (VITAMIN B-5) BRAIN BENEFITS

Pantothenic acid is required for energy, normal brain function, and fat metabolism. It is involved in the production of neurotransmitters, especially acetylcholine, which helps boost memory and regulate the autonomic nervous system. It is also important for boosting immunity.

Recommended Amount
50 to 200 mgs.

Top Kid-Friendly Pantothenic Acid Foods
Though pantothenic acid is readily available in the diet, it is not all that easy to get in the elimination stages of the diet for kids with a brain imbalance because some of the richest sources are the foods you will be eliminating: wheat, legumes, eggs, corn, and yogurt. Pantothenic acid is also abundant in other foods, however, especially all varieties of meats. These are the foods to look for:

- Avocado
- Banana
- Cabbage
- Collards
- Meats (all varieties)
- Poultry
- Prunes
- Shiitake mushrooms
- Spinach
- Squash
- Sunflower seeds

FOLATE BRAIN BENEFITS
Folate is crucial to proper brain function and plays an important role in emotional health and mental well-being. It aids in the production of DNA and RNA, the body's genetic material, and is particularly important during the rapid growth periods of infancy, childhood, and adolescence. This vitamin is also important for optimal nerve function. Along with vitamins B-6 and B-12, folate helps reduce homocysteine levels, which are implicated in FDS. Studies show that behavioral and emotional symptoms escalate in children who have low folate levels.

As every mother knows, folate deficiency during pregnancy is responsible for the neural birth defects spina bifida and cleft palate, which have greatly decreased, thanks to the widespread use of prenatal vitamins during pregnancy.

Recommended Amount

500 to 1,000 mgs, taken as supplemental folic acid. About 25 percent of people with autism have difficulty absorbing folate. For them, 500 to 1,000 mcg of 5 methyltetrahydrofolate is recommended.

Top Kid-Friendly Folate Foods

Because folate is such an important brain nutrient, you want to make sure to feed your child an abundance of high-folate foods. Eating naturally occurring folate through foods has been found to be better at reducing homocysteine than ingesting folic acid supplements. The best food sources, however—beans, lentils, oranges, and wheat—are common food sensitivities, and for this reason they are not recommended for kids with a brain imbalance. But folate is available in an abundance of plant foods, another reason to urge your kids to eat their vegetables! Reach for these high-folate foods:

- Asparagus
- Avocado
- Broccoli
- Brussels sprouts
- Carrots
- Cauliflower
- Collards and other dark leafy greens (spinach, romaine, mustard greens, etc.)
- Mango
- Nuts (all varieties, especially almonds)
- Seeds (all varieties, especially flaxseeds and sunflower seeds)

BIOTIN BRAIN BENEFITS

Although we need biotin in only small amounts, the brain is more dependent on this nutrient than any other organ. It is important to maintaining a healthy nervous system regulating gene expression.

Recommended Amount
12 to 20 mcg.

Top Kid-Friendly Biotin Foods
Like many of the other B vitamins, biotin is found in a lot of the foods that you'll want to avoid when starting out on the diet for kids with a brain imbalance—eggs, milk, legumes, and tomatoes. Other good sources of biotin include:

- Almonds
- Berries
- Cauliflower
- Dark chocolate
- Halibut
- Onions
- Peanut butter (organic)
- Salmon
- Sweet potatoes
- Swiss chard
- Walnuts

VITAMIN C BRAIN BENEFITS
Here's the reason vitamin C is so important to your child's brain health: Levels of this powerful antioxidant are typically fifteen times higher in the brain than in other parts of the body. Its contributions to healthy brain function are numerous. Among them: It is important in manufacturing the brain's most important neurotransmitters, including acetylcholine, dopamine, and norepinephrine; it is essential to regulating special receptors in the brain that modulate the rapid communication between cells in the brain; and it is involved in gene expression during brain development.

Several studies have found that many children with ADHD do not have an adequate supply of vitamin C in the blood. On the opposite end of the spectrum, one study found that higher than normal levels of vitamin C increased student IQ scores by an average of 5 points. In a study on children with autism, supplemental vitamin C reduced the severity of symptoms and improved sensory-motor-skill scores.

If your child has allergies or is prone to colds, extra vitamin C can help improve resistance. Though a true vitamin C deficiency is rare, studies show there is a risk for children with severe food avoidance behaviors.

Recommended Amount
500 mgs as a supplement twice a day.

Top Kid-Friendly Vitamin C Foods
The major sources of vitamin C are citrus foods, especially orange juice, tomatoes, and tomato juice, which are all potential sensitivity foods for kids with FDS. However, vitamin C is abundant in *a lot* of fruits and vegetables, such as these:

- Bell peppers
- Berries
- Brussels sprouts
- Cantaloupe
- Cauliflower
- Kiwi
- Leafy greens, especially kale
- Mango
- Papaya
- Pineapple
- Potatoes

VITAMIN D BRAIN BENEFITS
It's turning out that the decades-old push to prevent skin cancer is resulting in some unintended consequences, most notably the rising rate of vitamin D deficiency, which is believed to be associated with a higher risk of a variety of diseases, including those involved in impaired brain func-

tion. One study that reviewed the literature on vitamin D deficiency and autism stated that "vitamin D deficiency during pregnancy and childhood is a widespread and growing epidemic."

In my book *Autism: The Scientific Truth About Preventing, Diagnosing, and Treating Autism Spectrum Disorders—and What Parents Can Do Now*, I point to the growing body of research showing that a vitamin D deficiency in parents increases the risk of having a child with autism. So it is no stretch of the imagination to realize the important role vitamin D plays in healthy brain development.

We are learning more and more every day about the association between the "sunshine vitamin" and brain health. For example, we know that there are receptors for vitamin D throughout the central nervous system and in the hippocampus, which is involved in memory. We also know that vitamin D activates and deactivates enzymes in the brain and cerebrospinal fluid that are involved in neurotransmitter synthesis and nerve growth. And more and more studies are showing an association between vitamin D stores and healthy cognitive function.

In one study vitamin D levels in teens and young adults with autism spectrum disorders were "significantly lower" than those without the condition. Research suggest that vitamin D's anti-inflammatory action may make supplementation an effective means of fighting conditions on the autism spectrum.

Recommended Amount
2,000 to 5,000 IU as supplemental D-3.

Top Kid-Friendly Vitamin D Foods
There are many foods fortified with vitamin D—milk being the major source. Since your child may have a casein sensitivity, however, you need to depend on other foods to help protect against a deficiency. You aren't likely to achieve the recommended amount each day without supplements in the form of vitamin D-3, as dietary vitamin D is found mostly in dairy, eggs, and fortified orange juice. These are some nondairy sources of vitamin D:

- Flounder
- Fortified cereals
- Fortified almond milk
- Halibut
- Liver
- Pork
- Salmon
- Shiitake mushrooms
- Trout
- Tuna

VITAMIN E BRAIN BENEFITS

Vitamin E is a powerful antioxidant that protects the brain from the daily barrage of free radicals and oxidative stress. Some studies suggest that children with lower concentrations of vitamin E have more behavior problems, tempter tantrums, learning problems, and sleep disturbances than children with higher levels. Studies show that when combined with selenium, vitamin E helps improve mood and cognitive function.

Recommended Amount
400 IU, taken as a mixed tocopherol.

Top Kid-Friendly Vitamin E Foods
Vitamin E is not abundant in a lot of foods, which is why supplementation can be important for your child. Look to these sources:

- Avocado
- Broccoli
- Nuts, especially almonds and their oil
- Olive oil and other vegetable oils
- Peanut butter
- Pumpkin
- Spinach
- Shrimp
- Sunflower seeds and their oil

CALCIUM BRAIN BENEFITS

We already know that calcium is important to growing bones, but it has an impact on brain health too. This mineral is so involved in every phase of brain cell development that at least one study suggests that calcium deficiency during pregnancy increases the risk of autism and other developmental conditions. The study, reported in the journal *Progress in Brain Research*, demonstrates that the calcium signaling that occurs during the growth and strengthening of synaptic connections in the brain helps to optimize emerging networks to perform their specific functions. Calcium deficiency is common in autistic children. When taken as a supplement, calcium can have a calming effect on behavior.

Recommended Amount

1,000 to 2,000 mgs, taken as calcium carbonate liquid or chewable tablets.

Top Kid-Friendly Calcium Foods

Our best food sources of this important mineral are milk and other dairy products, which very well could be a problem for a child with FDS. This may mean supplementation is necessary. While everyone thinks "dairy" when it comes to getting calcium, there are other foods you can turn to for the mineral. These are all good sources:

- Almonds
- Blackstrap molasses
- Bok choy
- Collards
- Figs
- Iceberg lettuce
- Kale
- Salmon
- Sesame seeds
- Turnip greens

MAGNESIUM BRAIN BENEFITS

Magnesium is not a mineral people generally pay much attention to, but that's not the case where I'm concerned. I value it because it is involved with virtually every function in the body. It supports a healthy immune system and helps prevent inflammation. It nourishes and calms the central nervous system and helps the body fight stress. It is also a common deficiency in children with ADHD and autism. Studies show that supplementation can help alleviate hyperactivity, irritability, and sleep disturbances in children with neurodevelopmental disorders.

Recommended Amount

200 to 600 mgs, taken as supplemental magnesium chloride or magnesium citrate.

Top Kid-Friendly Magnesium Foods

Though supplementation is warranted for many children with a brain imbalance, it is still important to eat magnesium-rich foods, because 50 percent more of the mineral is absorbed from foods than through supplements. While two of the best sources are whole grains and soy foods, the food chain offers us a wide variety of other sources of magnesium. Try these:

- Avocado
- Banana
- Brown rice
- Dark chocolate
- Dried figs
- Nuts, all varieties
- Pumpkin seeds, as well as other seeds
- Salmon
- Spinach and other green leafy vegetables
- Squash

ZINC BRAIN BENEFITS

Zinc is a trace mineral important to optimizing brain function. How important? A review of environmental factors related to autism spectrum disorders found that a zinc deficiency has multiple adverse effects on the developing brain. In one study, researchers at Duke University Medical Center and the Massachusetts Institute of Technology used a chemical that binds with zinc to eliminate it from the brains of test mice. They found that in the absence of the mineral, communication between neurons was significantly diminished. In another study, test animals with a zinc deficiency displayed abnormal autism-related behaviors, such as impaired vocalization and hyperactivity.

Specifically, zinc is needed for the development and maintenance of the brain, GI tract, immune system, and adrenal glands. It is associated with building memory and cognitive abilities. According to DAN (Defeat Autism Now!), zinc is deficient in 90 percent of children with an autism spectrum disorder.

Recommended Amount
10 mgs.

Top Kid-Friendly Zinc Foods
Oysters are by far are the major source of dietary zinc, but I've yet to meet a child who will dare give them a try! Instead, go for these kid-friendlier foods:

- Almonds
- Beef
- Cashews
- Chicken
- Cocoa and dark chocolate
- Flounder
- Mushrooms
- Shrimp
- Spinach

ZINC, COPPER, AND ASD

When it comes to brain health, zinc and copper are inter-related. When zinc levels go down, copper levels go up. One study of 318 people with autism spectrum disorders found that 85 percent of them had an abnormally high copper-to zinc-ratio. Since copper is a mineral often found in excess in kids with a brain imbalance, do not give your child a multivitamin that contains any copper.

SELENIUM BRAIN BENEFITS

Selenium is an important antioxidant trace mineral essential to the development and functioning of areas of the brain involved in thinking and emotional regulation. It is also important in preventing and reversing oxidative damage in the brain. Low selenium levels have been linked to irritability and decreased cognitive functioning and clarity. Low selenium levels are also common in children with ADHD.

Recommended Amount
100 mcg.

Top Kid-Friendly Selenium Foods
Though it is readily available in meats, fish, grains, vegetables, and fruits, the quality and quantity of this mineral are largely dependent on the amount found in the earth and water where food grows or animals feed. Some of the most readily available sources are believed to be sardines, herring, and anchovies, foods not found in the daily diets of many kids *or* adults. However, you can help boost your kids' selenium levels by serving these foods:

- Beef
- Brazil and other nuts
- Brown rice

- Chicken breast
- Garlic
- Mushrooms
- Mustard and mustard seeds
- Onion
- Rice bran
- Shrimp
- Tuna

MANGANESE BRAIN BENEFITS

Manganese is a trace mineral very important to the normal functioning of the brain and the central nervous system. It is particularly beneficial to children with FDS because of its positive effects on the digestive system. It helps encourage smooth functioning of the digestive tract, improves fat metabolism, reduces issues involved in constipation and bowel discomfort, and helps turn food into energy efficiently.

Recommended Amount
200 to 400 mgs.

Top Kid-Friendly Manganese Foods
While soy and wheat are rich sources of manganese, this trace mineral can also be found in these foods:

- Banana
- Beets
- Blackstrap molasses
- Brown rice
- Carrots
- Coconut
- Dried figs
- Green beans
- Hazelnuts
- Mustard greens and other green leafy vegetables

POTASSIUM BRAIN BENEFITS

Potassium helps carry oxygen to the brain and keep the brain and nerves working at their best. It also helps carry impulses from the brain to the large muscles. Without an adequate supply of potassium, it is almost impossible to think clearly.

Recommended Amount

3,000 to 4,000 mgs. Excessive levels can interfere with normal heart and nervous system function.

Top Kid-Friendly Potassium Foods

Potassium is plentiful in the food supply of a well-balanced diet. It's in all meats, fish, and chicken and in these foods:

- Baking potato in its jacket
- Banana
- Blackstrap molasses
- Carrot juice
- Dried apricots
- Leafy greens
- Mushrooms
- Squash
- Sweet potatoes
- Swiss chard

MOLYBDENUM BRAIN BENEFITS

Molybdenum is a trace mineral that fights inflammation and autoimmune diseases, which are common in FDS. It also helps activate enzymes for removing toxins from the brain and body.

Recommended Amount

17 to 34 mcgs, depending on age.

Top Kid-Friendly Molybdenum Foods

Most of the foods containing molybdenum are the beans and grains that are a source of sensitivity in many children with FDS. However, you can also find it in these foods:

- Almonds
- Brown rice
- Cashews
- Peanut butter
- Pineapple
- Pumpkin seeds
- Spinach

ESSENTIAL FATTY ACIDS

These nutrients are considered "essential" because they are required for human health in general and brain function in particular. They function as constituents of cell membranes, helping to relay signals from outside the cells to their interiors. They are crucially important to brain development during pregnancy and after birth. They are also important in a Brain Balance Program because studies are revealing a link between shortages of essential fatty acids and the rising incidence of neurological childhood disorders. Several studies show that the physical symptoms of ADHD are similar to symptoms found in EFA-deficienct animals and humans. While we need *all* essential fatty acids in the diet, these are the ones you should focus on:

Omega-3 Fatty Acids

Omega-3 fatty acids are particularly important because they are consistently found to be deficient in children with autism spectrum disorders. Although only a few studies have been conducted on omega-3 deficiency and autism, the results are consistent. One study found omega-3 deficiency in nearly 100 percent of children with an autism spectrum disorder, and another found it in 90 percent of children studied. In addition, studies suggest that approximately 40 percent of boys with ADHD do not get adequate amounts of fatty acids in the diet.

Recommended Amount
1,000 to 3,000 mgs.

Top Kid-Friendly Omega-3 Foods
Omega-3s are found most notably in the oils of fatty fish and seeds, particularly flaxseed. These are some of the best sources:

- Brussels sprouts
- Flaxseed
- Nuts and nut oils, especially walnuts
- Salmon
- Shrimp
- Tuna
- Winter squash

Alpha Lipoic Acid
ALA, as it is commonly known, is the synthetic version of lipoic acid, a type of fatty acid occurring naturally in the body that has a protective effect on the brain and central nervous system. As a supplement, it increases insulin sensitivity and works with B vitamins to help convert foods to energy. It also aids in restoring levels of some vitamins, such as C and E, and is used in the body to break down carbohydrates. In one study supplementation with ALA in the form of flaxseed oil showed "significant improvement" in reducing the symptoms of ADHD and improving scores on the hyperactivity scale.

Recommended Amount
200 to 600 mgs.

Top Kid-Friendly Alpha Lipoic Acid Foods
ALA occurs naturally in only a small number of foods, most specifically organ meats, such as kidneys (a food not popular with fussy eaters), as well as these foods:

- Broccoli
- Brussels sprouts
- Liver
- Potatoes
- Spinach
- Swiss chard

DIGESTIVE ENZYMES

One of the major challenges associated with FDS is the poor digestion that goes along with a leaky gut. The digestive tracts of most of these children do not break down food properly. This is largely due to the fact that they have fewer secretions—mainly hydrochloric acid and enzymes—in the digestive tract that are needed to chemically break down and digest food so it can cross the tight junctions in the stomach and intestines and be absorbed. We find that supplementing the diet with digestive enzymes is essential in correcting the problem. Once the brain starts to regulate these secretions better, the use of these digestive acid supplements can be stopped.

Recommended Amount

There is no exact dosage recommended for digestive enzymes. I suggest starting with the smallest dosage and increasing it while watching for changes in digestive discomfort.

Coenzyme Q10 Brain Benefits

CoQ10, as it is commonly called, is a naturally occurring vitamin-like substance found throughout the body in high concentrations. It helps defend and repair cells from oxidative stress. It is required by all cells, including brain cells, to make energy. Research shows that children with a brain imbalance, particularly those with autism, are more vulnerable to the oxidative stress that damages and ages cells. Low concentrations of CoQ10 cause low energy in the body and the brain.

For the first time in 2014, researchers found that supplementing children's diets with a nutritional form of CoQ10 resulted in a marked decrease in symptoms. After three month, the researchers reported a 42 percent improvement in interactive children's games; a 17 percent reduction in food rejection; a 21 percent improvement in verbal communication; and a 12 percent improvement in communication with parents.

Recommended Amount
90 to 100 mgs.

Top Kid-Friendly CoQ10 Foods
CoQ10 exists in small amounts in a variety of foods, but it is most plentiful in meat, poultry, fish, and oils. You can also find CoQ10 in:

- Broccoli
- Canola oil
- Cauliflower
- Spinach
- Sweet potatoes

PART II

Recipes from Our Staff and Guest Chefs

Chapter 6
Start-Smart Breakfasts

In most busy households, breakfast is more about store-bought, get-'em-out-the-door-fast cereals, waffles, and pancakes rather than whole foods made from scratch. That's understandable, of course, but not always a good choice in Brain Balance households. Many quick-fix packaged breakfasts are filled with additives and preservatives that can trigger food sensitivities in children. And, of course, there's gluten, which is a problem for most kids with a leaky gut.

All children need a nutritious breakfast to stimulate the brain into learning mode, so don't sell this meal short. Ideally, it should contain a healthy balance of protein, healthy monounsaturated fats, and complex carbohydrates, potent macronutrients that are crucial for cognition. It's the perfect way to start the day.

Just because you're going gluten free and avoiding prepackaged food does not mean breakfast has to be a challenge. Make-your-own breakfasts need not be extravagant or time consuming. You also don't need to offer your kids something different every day. I suggest you try as many of the following as appeal to you. When you find one or a few recipes that your kids love, stick with them. All of these recipes are easy to prepare, and most of the cereals you find here can be prepared ahead of time and in big batches.

HOW TO USE THESE RECIPES

Virtually all the recipes in this book avoid gluten and casein, and the majority of them are free of the foods on the 10 Most Wanted List—those most likely to cause a sensitivity. However, a child can be sensitive to almost any food. Avoid using any recipe that includes an ingredient that your elimination diet reveals your child could be sensitive to. Or, if possible, exclude it from the recipe. You can start using these recipes once you are sure the sensitivity is a thing of the past.

INSTANT COCONUT-CINNAMON BREAKFAST CEREAL

Connie Portman, nutrition counselor at the Brain Balance center in Tulsa, Oklahoma, developed this ready-to-cook hot cereal as a nutritious substitute for store-bought varieties. The kids at the center love it! You can double or triple it depending on the size of your family and how frequently you'll serve it. Serve it with casein-free milk.

Makes 3 cups

1 cup chia seeds
1 cup ground flax meal
1 cup unsweetened shredded coconut
1 teaspoon ground cinnamon

Combine all of the ingredients together and store in an airtight container.

Note: To make a single serving of this cereal, place ½ cup of cereal in a bowl and add ⅔ cup simmering water. Stir and let stand for 3 to 4 minutes. Add 2 tablespoons of almond or rice milk and 1 tablespoon of agave nectar.

GRAIN-FREE GRANOLA

There are no worries about gluten when you mix your own granola. Thanks for this recipe goes to Kristen Davidson, nutrition coach at the Brain Balance Achievement Center in Overland Park and greater Kansas City in Kansas. Serve it with fruit and your choice of milk.

Makes about 5 cups

 2 cups raw, unsalted sunflower seeds
 2 cups raw, unsalted pumpkin seeds
 1 cup unsweetened shredded coconut
 1 cup pecan pieces
 ½ cup coconut oil, melted
 ½ cup honey
 1 tablespoon ground cinnamon
 ½ teaspoon sea salt

1. Preheat the oven to 325°F.

2. In a large bowl combine the seeds, coconut, and pecan pieces.

3. In a small bowl combine the melted oil, honey, cinnamon, and salt. Mix well. Pour the liquid ingredients over the dry ingredients, stirring with a wooden spoon to make sure all the dry ingredients are coated.

4. Line two baking sheets with parchment paper. Divide the mixture between the two baking sheets, spreading it around so the pieces do not stick together, and bake in the preheated oven for 25 to 30 minutes. Cool for 30 minutes and store in an airtight container.

DR. ED'S ALMOND CEREAL[1]

This is a popular breakfast with the kids who attend the Brain Balance Achievement Centers in Peachtree City, Roswell, and Suwannee, Georgia. It is a highly nutritious, low-glycemic meal that will give your child energy throughout the day without sugar spikes or crashes, says center director Dr. Ed Finucan. If your child is not dairy sensitive, use organic whole milk. Otherwise opt for a nut milk. Almond is okay, though it might make the meal taste too almondy. You can try other nut milks, such as hazelnut and macadamia, which can be found at some higher-end markets, such as Whole Foods. This recipe makes one generous serving, but feel free

---

1 If your child is sensitive to apple, eliminate it and substitute it with another fruit.

to increase the amount to fit your family's need. Adjust the fruit to your liking.

Makes 1 serving

½ cup raw, unsalted almonds
¼ cup unsweetened shredded coconut or 1 packet Living Fuel Coco-Chia
1 teaspoon unsweetened cocoa powder
1 to 2 tablespoons melted coconut oil
10 raisins
½ apple, diced
1 cup almond milk, coconut milk, or unsweetened rice milk or regular milk

1. Put the almonds and coconut in a blender and grind to the consistency of a fine powder, or coarser, if desired.

2. Empty into a bowl and mix in the cocoa powder and coconut oil.

3. Add the raisins and apple, then pour on the milk. Serve cold or heat in the microwave and serve warm.

Note: Do not heat on the stovetop, as it will change the consistency.

GO ORGANIC WHENEVER POSSIBLE

Brain Balance nutritionists and parents know the importance of going organic in order to make sure the food they feed their children is as pure, natural, and chemical free as possible. These days organic produce can be found in most mainstream supermarkets. It may cost a little extra, but the feedback we get from families is that it is well worth it in helping to overcome their kids' food sensitivities and nutritional issues.

To this end, we recommend buying only organic fruits, vegetables, grains, spices, herbs, and sugar substitutes (agave nectars and honey) when preparing these recipes and preparing other foods at home. We do not specify organic in the ingredient lists, as we want you to consider it understood. Look for the words "natural," "organic," and "gluten free" when buying ingredients for these recipes.

SLOW-COOKER BROWN RICE PORRIDGE[2]

This morning cereal should rival most any kid's off-the-shelf favorite, says Jennifer Fugo, founder of glutenfreeschool.com and author of *The Savvy Gluten-Free Shopper*. This is one of her favorite gluten-free breakfasts, and it has a natural sweetness children love. This recipe makes a big batch that will keep well in the refrigerator all week long. All you need to do each morning is zap it in the microwave. It can also be frozen in single-serve containers. "Make sure to use short-grain rice," says Jennifer. "It just does not work with long-grain rice." For a protein boost, add one-half serving size of vanilla protein powder.

Makes 6 servings

1 cup short-grain brown rice, rinsed
5 cups water
2 large Granny Smith apples or 1 large Gala apple, cored and cubed
¼ cup raisins
¼ cup unsweetened shredded coconut
½ teaspoon pumpkin pie spice
¼ teaspoon ground cinnamon
Pinch sea salt

Combine all of the ingredients in a slow cooker set on low, cover, and cook for about 8 hours.

Variation: For an even creamier breakfast, stir in a tablespoon of natural nut butter just before serving.

---

2 This recipe contains apples, so do not use it if you find your child is sensitive to apples.

COCONUT MILLET WITH AROMATIC SPICES[3]

This warming breakfast cereal was created for the Brain Balance community by Christie Korth, Brain Balance corporate director of nutrition and award-winning author of *The IBD Healing Plan and Recipe Book*. The feedback has been terrific! She recommends using whole millet and grinding it in a coffee grinder or food processor. Or, you can put the millet in a paper or plastic bag and crush it with a rolling pin. If this seems like too much work, use prepared millet that is already ground. Read the package to make sure there are no unwanted additives.

Makes 2 to 3 servings

½ cup whole millet or Bob's Red Mill preground millet
1½ cups water
¼ cup grated unsweetened coconut
1 cup unsweetened applesauce
Pinch sea salt
½ teaspoon ground cinnamon
Pinch freshly grated or ground nutmeg
½ teaspoon ground cardamom

1. Toast the millet in a dry skillet over medium-low heat, tossing constantly, until fragrant and slightly golden-brown. Grind the millet in a coffee grinder or food processor, using short pulses so it does not turn into a paste. If using packaged ground millet, skip this step.

2. Bring the water to a boil in a medium saucepan. Add the ground millet, coconut, applesauce, salt, cinnamon, nutmeg, and cardamom. Immediately reduce the heat to low and cover. Simmer for 15 minutes, or until the cereal is tender, checking halfway through cooking to make sure the water hasn't all been absorbed. Add more water if necessary.

---

3 This recipe contains apples, so do not use it if you find that your child is sensitive to apples.

GLUTEN-FREE GRAINS

You can never be too careful when shopping for gluten-free items, especially when it comes to buying grains. Consider bulk bins in the supermarket off limits, recommends Jennifer Fugo, founder of Gluten Free School, an interactive website (glutenfreeschool.com) and author of *The Savvy Gluten-Free Shopper.* Cross contamination is much too easy.

"Unbeknownst to you, the store may have put your naturally gluten-free items in a bin that has formerly stored wheat," she cautions, "or the wheat flour in a container up higher could slowly settle downwards through the containers and end up in the 'gluten-free' bin you are buying from."

When buying in bulk, look for larger quantities of grains prepackaged by companies that clearly test and mark their products "certified gluten free."

BANANA-BERRY CEREAL

Homemade doesn't get any faster than this! This idea is courtesy of Janeil Swarthout, Ph.D., executive director of the Brain Balance Achievement Center in Fresno-Clovis, California.

Makes 1 serving

1 ripe banana, chopped
¼ cup fresh strawberries
2 tablespoons slivered or sliced almonds
1 cup almond or coconut milk

Put the bananas, berries, and almonds in a cereal bowl and add the milk.

CHERRY-BANANA BUCKWHEAT PUDDING

Don't let the name of the grain throw you. Buckwheat and wheat are from different botanical families—and buckwheat is gluten free. This pudding can be served for breakfast or dessert and made in advance, says creator Christie Korth, corporate director of nutrition for Brain Balance. Simply store in the refrigerator and reheat in a saucepan. You may want to add a tad of the butter substitute Earth Balance spread while reheating if the pudding becomes too thick or gloppy. This will assist in its return to a smoother, creamier consistency.

Makes 4 servings

1 tablespoon Earth Balance spread
1¼ teaspoons pumpkin pie spice
2½ cups filtered water
1 cup buckwheat
¼ tablespoon sea salt
1 cup vanilla almond milk
3 tablespoons blueberry agave nectar, plus more if needed
¼ cup dried cherries
⅓ cup coarsely chopped walnuts, toasted
1 teaspoon pure vanilla extract
1 teaspoon orange zest
1 ripe banana, sliced on a diagonal

1. Set a heavy 3-quart saucepan over medium-high heat. Add the Earth Balance. As it melts, stir in the pumpkin pie spice.

2. Gradually stir in the water (watch out for splattering), buckwheat, and salt. Bring to a boil over high heat. Lower the heat slightly, cover, and boil over medium-high heat, stirring occasionally, until most of the water is absorbed, 5 to 8 minutes.

3. Stir in the milk, agave nectar, and cherries and return to a boil. Cook, uncovered, over medium heat, stirring frequently to prevent the grains from sticking to the bottom, until the buckwheat is tender (it will al-

ways remain a little chewy) and the pudding develops a porridge-like texture, 6 to 8 minutes.

4. Remove from the heat. The pudding will continue to thicken as it cools. Add more agave, if needed. Stir in the walnuts and vanilla.

Serve in small bowls, warm or at room temperature. Garnish each portion with orange zest and banana slices.

RICE PUDDING

Get your children off to a great start with the terrific combination of carbohydrates, calcium, and protein from this breakfast pudding, says Tulsa center's Connie Portman. It's the perfect warm-'em-up for chilly school mornings.

Makes 4 servings

2 cups cooked brown rice
1⅔ cups nondairy milk, such as unsweetened almond or rice milk
3 tablespoons agave nectar
½ teaspoon ground cinnamon
½ teaspoon pure vanilla extract
3 tablespoons chia seeds

Combine the rice, milk, and agave nectar in a medium saucepan and cook over medium heat until bubbly, 8 to 10 minutes. Remove from the heat and add the cinnamon, vanilla, and chia seeds. Let sit for 5 minutes. Spoon into parfait glasses and serve.

STRAWBERRY-BANANA SMOOTHIE[4]

Smoothies are a great way to literally pour nutrition down your kid's throat in the morning, says Christie Korth. If berries aren't in season, substitute frozen, but do not thaw, she says. For addi-

---

4 Citrus is a common food sensitivity, so don't use this recipe if you find that your child is intolerant to citrus.

tional nutrition, add vitamin powders to this drink, such as a packet of vitamin C or zinc. This smoothie is an immune system booster, good for when your kid has a cold.

Makes 2 servings

    2 ripe medium bananas
    2 cups hulled strawberries, fresh or frozen
    1 to 2 cups orange juice, fresh squeezed if possible
    Juice of one lime
    1 tablespoon honey
    1 tablespoon ground flaxseed (optional)

In a blender, combine the bananas, strawberries, 1 cup of the orange juice, lime juice, honey, and flaxseed, if using. Blend, adding additional orange juice a little at a time if necessary, until the smoothie is thick but pourable.

CHOCOLATE-ALMOND SMOOTHIE

"This smoothie tastes like a chocolate milkshake, so kids love it," says my sister-in-law Susan Melillo, who offers this breakfast idea to families at the Brain Balance Achievement Center in Wake Forest, North Carolina, where she is the executive director. "It is an easy and tasty way to get protein first thing in the morning and helps prevent hunger for hours." Add more or less cocoa, depending on how chocolaty your child likes it. If your child's nutritional profile allows it, you can substitute peanut butter for the almond butter.

Makes 1 serving

    ¾ cup almond milk
    15 ice cubes
    ½ teaspoon pure vanilla extract
    1 to 2 tablespoons unsweetened cocoa powder
    ⅓ ripe banana
    1 to 2 teaspoons almond butter

Put all of the ingredients in a blender and blend on high until smooth, about 15 to 20 seconds.

CHERRY-WALNUT BREAKFAST LOAF

This is the ideal sweet gluten-free bread for families who are running off in different directions in the morning and can't always take the time for a sit-down breakfast. It's easy to stuff in the backpacks of kids who like to nibble their breakfast on the way to school. And it also makes a great after-school snack. The kids at the Huntington Beach (California) Brain Balance Achievement Center rated it high for its "sweet and refreshing" taste, says cognitive coach Hadley McGregor. To maintain its freshness, keep the bread refrigerated. It will keep for about a week. The small amount of orange juice should not affect a child with a sensitivity.

Makes 1 loaf

1 cup raw, unrefined sugar
1¼ teaspoons baking powder
½ teaspoon baking soda
2 cups Donna's GF All-Purpose Flour (page 188) or store-bought
   flour (rice or tapioca flour works well)
½ teaspoon sea salt
¼ teaspoon ground allspice
½ cup rice milk
¼ cup freshly squeezed orange juice
¼ cup canola oil
1 teaspoon pure vanilla extract
1 cup pitted fresh or frozen cherries, halved (if frozen, make sure
   they are well drained)
½ cup chopped walnuts

1. Preheat the oven to 325°F.

2. In a large mixing bowl combine the sugar, baking powder, baking soda, flour, salt, and allspice. Using a spoon or whisk, gradually mix in the rice milk, orange juice, oil, and vanilla extract. Fold in the cherries and walnuts.

3. Pour the batter into a lightly greased 9 x 5-inch loaf pan. Bake for 1 hour, or until a toothpick inserted in the center comes out clean.

4. Let the bread cool for about 15 to 20 minutes.

PUMPKIN PIE MUFFINS

It's not hard to sell kids on morning muffins when you say "pumpkin pie." These muffins—courtesy of the Brain Balance Achievement Center in Midlothian, Virginia, and the centers in Cary and Chapel Hill, North Carolina—are enriched with flaxseeds, an excellent source of omega-3 fatty acids. They are so popular in director Rebecca Jackson's household that she doubles the recipe and sends them along with school lunches or serves them as an after-school snack. If you follow suit, she recommends creaming the mixture in two batches.

Makes 1 dozen muffins

½ cup almond or other nut butter
One and a half 15-ounce cans unsweetened pumpkin puree
2 large eggs or equivalent of Donna's Egg Replacer (page 184)
¾ cup honey
1 cup gluten-free oats or cooked quinoa
¼ cup ground flaxseeds
2 teaspoons ground cinnamon
1 teaspoon ground nutmeg
1 teaspoon ground cloves
2 teaspoons pure vanilla extract
1 teaspoon baking soda
½ cup dark chocolate chips or raisins

1. Preheat the oven to 375°F.

2. Put all of the ingredients except for the chocolate chips or raisins in a blender or food processor and process on high until the oats are broken down and the batter is smooth and creamy. Fold in the chocolate chips or raisins.

3. Spray a muffin tin with nonstick spray. Fill the cups evenly ⅔ to ¾ full with the batter.

4. Bake for 10 to 12 minutes, or until a toothpick inserted in the center comes out clean. Cool and store in the refrigerator. They will keep for about a week.

BIRTHDAY BLUEBERRY MUFFINS

A little bit of potato starch adds a dense cake-like consistency to these muffins, and the glycerin, available at stores selling organic ingredients, helps sweeten and hold these muffins together. "My daughter, who has a lot of food sensitivities, asks for these every year for her birthday breakfast," says Stacey Gadbois, who teaches parents how to cook for food sensitivities at the Brain Balance Achievement Center in Virginia Beach, Virginia. Stacey says most egg replacers do not work well with this recipe so she recommends using real eggs if they are allowed on your child's diet.

Makes 1 dozen muffins

2 large eggs
4 tablespoons melted clarified butter or ghee
½ tablespoon vegetable glycerin
1 teaspoon pure vanilla extract
½ cup xylitol
2½ cups natural almond flour
⅛ cup potato starch
1 teaspoon baking soda
1 teaspoon ground cinnamon
¼ teaspoon sea salt
1 cup fresh blueberries

1. Preheat the oven to 350°F.

2. In a large bowl cream the eggs, clarified butter, vegetable glycerin, vanilla, and xylitol with an electric mixer on low speed.

3. In a separate bowl combine the almond flour, potato starch, baking soda, cinnamon, and salt. Add the dry ingredients to the wet mixture and mix on low speed until combined. Fold in the blueberries.

4. Put liners into a muffin tin. Pour the batter evenly into the tins ⅔ to ¾ full. Bake for 25 minutes, or until a toothpick inserted in the center of the muffins comes out clean. If using egg replacer, cover the muffins with foil after baking for 25 minutes, and bake for an additional 10 to 15 minutes. Refrigerate after serving.

CLARIFYING BUTTER

Going casein free? Butter can still be included in the diet as long as you use clarified butter. Casein is a milk protein that is found in the foamy top you see on butter when it is melted. Remove the milk proteins from the butter through a process called "clarifying" and you end up with casein-free butter. Clarified butter is also sold as *ghee*.

To make clarified butter, put a pound of butter in a small ovenproof dish and place it in a 350°F oven until it is melted, about 12 minutes. Be sure you do not burn the butter. Remove it from the oven and let it stand for 5 minutes.

Skim the foam from the top with a large spoon. Slowly pour in a storage container, discarding the milk solids in the bottom of the dish. You'll lose about one quarter of the butter you started with. Clarified butter will keep refrigerated in a sealed container for about a month.

Chapter 7
All Souped Up

To me, nothing says family comfort food like a bowl of homemade soup simmering on the stove. We love soups at Brain Balance because they are such a tasty and satisfying way to get more vegetables in a child's diet. And they offer so many advantages.

For one, soup is gentle on a sensitive gastrointestinal tract. It's a great way to introduce new foods into your finicky eater's diet. Just puree onions, celery, and carrots into chicken broth when you are making soup, and you have just added *three* new vegetables to your child's diet without him even knowing it!

Making soup is convenient for busy families—a pot can go a long, long way. Plus, it freezes well. And, soup is quite versatile. It can be served as dinner or lunch. Best of all, you can put it in a thermos and send it along as a school lunch. Pair it with a green salad and a piece of fruit and you have a full meal loaded with nutrients.

PUREED VEGETABLE SOUP WITH A KICK

Rebecca Jackson—executive director for the Brain Balance Achievement Center in Midlothian, Virginia, and the centers in Cary and Chapel Hill, North Carolina—loves this recipe for its convenience. It tastes good warm or cold and goes to school nicely in a thermos. "Kale and zucchini are not things my kids typically eat, but when they're pureed in with everything else, they eat them in this soup without even realizing it!" she says.

Makes about 10 servings

2 onions, chopped
1 bunch kale, coarsely chopped
3 medium zucchini, coarsely chopped

3 medium carrots, peeled and coarsely chopped

2 cups broccoli florets

2 cups coarsely chopped butternut squash

Two 15-ounce cans chickpeas, drained and rinsed

1 quart water

One 15-ounce can full-fat coconut milk

8 cloves garlic, peeled and chopped

2 tablespoons chopped fresh ginger

1 tablespoon poultry seasoning

1 teaspoon ground cumin

1 teaspoon ground turmeric

1 teaspoon cayenne

1 bay leaf

Put all of the ingredients in a large stockpot and bring to a boil. Reduce the heat and simmer until the squash is soft, about 20 minutes. Remove the bay leaf and cool slightly. Puree in batches in a blender.

THAI SWEET-POTATO SOUP

"We serve this dish with no flatware, and the kids use crackers or bread as a 'spoon.' The novelty of that simple change makes eating this soup fun," says Rebecca Jackson. "It freezes well, so make a big batch."

Makes 8 to 10 servings

1 tablespoon coconut oil

1 small onion, coarsely chopped

2 teaspoons chopped garlic

3 cups gluten-free vegetable stock

4 large sweet potatoes, peeled and coarsely chopped

½ to 1 teaspoon red curry paste

Juice of 1 lime

1. Heat the oil in a large Dutch oven over medium heat. Add the onion and cook until soft, about 3 minutes. Add the garlic and cook for 1 minute. Stir in the stock and sweet potato.

2. Bring to a boil, reduce the heat to medium, cover, and cook for 15 minutes. Remove from the heat. Stir in the red curry paste and squeeze fresh lime juice into the mixture. Cool slightly. Puree in batches in a blender until smooth. Return to the pan and heat through.

CHICKEN-RICE SOUP

Parents at the Brain Balance Achievement Center in Tulsa, Oklahoma, like this soup because it is so easy to make. Pack it in a thermos for lunch or pair it with a green salad and fresh fruit for dinner. It makes a large batch and is freezable.

Makes 6 to 8 servings

2 cups cooked diced chicken
2 stalks celery, minced
½ cup diced yellow onion
2 cups uncooked brown basmati rice
8 cups water
2 tablespoons Better than Bouillon chicken base
½ teaspoon black pepper

Put all of the ingredients in a large stockpot. Bring to a boil, then turn down to a simmer for 20 minutes, or until the rice is soft. Or, add all of the ingredients to a slow cooker and cook on low for 4 to 6 hours.

CHICKEN-QUINOA SOUP[1]

Here's a more Brain Balance–friendly approach to chicken-rice soup. "Quinoa is the mother of all grains and is packed with lots of B vitamins, which help improve concentration, plus plenty of protein," says Brain Balance corporate nutritionist and recipe creator Christie Korth.

Makes 6 servings

---

1 Omit the beans if you determine that your child has a sensitivity to beans.

1 tablespoon olive oil
1 pound chicken breasts, cut into ¼-inch pieces
Sea salt and black pepper to taste
8 ounces white mushrooms, sliced
2 stalks celery, sliced thin
1 cup cooked quinoa
One 15-ounce can cannellini beans, drained and rinsed
4 cups unsalted chicken broth
3 tablespoons fresh lemon juice
¾ cup fresh flat-leaf parsley leaves

1. In a large pot heat the olive oil over medium-high heat. Add the chicken, season with salt and pepper, and cook, stirring occasionally, until just cooked through, about 5 minutes.

2. Add the mushrooms and celery and cook until the chicken is golden-brown, about 10 minutes.

3. Stir in the cooked quinoa, beans, broth, and lemon juice. Season with salt and pepper. Lower the heat and simmer until heated through. Stir in the parsley.

COCONUT CURRY SOUP[2]

This simple-to-make Asian soup is an example of how to use Lisa Carlson's Multipurpose Chicken (page 150). Lisa, director of the Brain Balance Achievement center in Minnetonka, Minnesota, says it's a family favorite. Sometimes she adds red or green bell peppers, if she has them on hand. Add more curry or coconut sugar to make it as spicy or as sweet as you like. It freezes well, so you can double or even triple a batch.

Makes 4 to 6 servings

---

2   Do not serve this recipe if you determine that your child is sensitive to tomatoes.

3 tablespoons red Thai curry paste

Two 14-ounce cans full-fat coconut milk

¼ cup coconut sugar

2 cups chicken stock

1 teaspoon Asian fish sauce

¾ cup diced fresh or canned tomatoes

3 carrots, peeled and sliced

1 cup snow peas or 1 cup frozen peas, frozen or thawed

4 ounces (½ package) rice noodles

1 cooked shredded chicken, such as Lisa's Multipurpose Chicken
(page 150)

1. Put the curry paste in a large soup pot or Dutch oven over medium-high heat and whisk in ¼ cup of the coconut milk and the coconut sugar until smooth. Add the remaining milk, the chicken stock, and fish sauce. Stir until combined and bring to a simmer.

2. Add the tomatoes, carrots, and peas and cook until tender, about 8 to 10 minutes. Add the noodles and chicken. Cook on medium heat until the noodles are tender, about 4 minutes.

Chapter 8
Dinner Delightful

Mom and Dad are not short-order cooks! This is a mantra for mealtime sanity. The biggest mistake parents make is feeding a food-fussy kid something other than what the rest of the household is eating. On the other hand, it's not fair to make kids eat food that doesn't suit their young palates, either. The happy medium is dinner entrées the entire family can enjoy. Sometimes all it takes is the right sell to get kids to bite . . . and bite again. Our Brain Balance nutritionists, families, and friends have become pros at concocting meals that make family dinners delightful.

LEMON-PEPPER CHICKEN-ON-A-STICK[1]

Rusty Hamlin, executive chef of Zac Brown Band's Eat and Greet concert venues, knows how to make crowd-pleasing food, and that extends right to the kids who tested this recipe. It was a big hit—they loved the idea of eating chicken right off the stick. Serve this with Rusty's Cajun Red Potato Fries (page 166) and Grilled Asparagus (page 178) for a complete meal.

Makes 6 servings

2 pounds boneless, skinless chicken breast
3 tablespoons olive oil
4 lemons, zested and juiced
2 tablespoons cracked black pepper
1½ tablespoons sea salt

---

1 Avoid this recipe if you determine that your child has a citrus sensitivity.

3 cloves garlic, minced

2 tablespoons chopped fresh basil

Twelve 10-inch bamboo skewers, soaked in water

1. Preheat your grill.

2. Wash the chicken, pat it dry, and cut it into 1-inch-wide strips. Put the olive oil, lemon juice and zest, black pepper, salt, garlic, and basil in a large bowl. Add the chicken strips and marinate in the refrigerator for 1 hour.

3. Remove the chicken from the refrigerator and bring it to room temperature. Loosely skewer the chicken pieces onto the bamboo skewers, ribbon style. You do not want to crowd them. Put the chicken on the grill at high heat and grill for 3 minutes. Turn and grill for 3 minutes more, or until cooked through.

BROILED TANDOORI-SPICED SALMON WITH AVOCADO-SPINACH QUINOA

These ingredients make for a super-nutritious meal, courtesy of Zac Brown's personal chef, Collins Woods.

Makes 4 servings

FOR THE QUINOA

1 cup uncooked quinoa

1½ cups chicken broth

½ teaspoon garlic powder

1 avocado, diced

3 cups roughly chopped fresh spinach

Sea salt to taste

FOR THE SALMON

Four 6-ounce wild skinless salmon fillets, deboned

Sea salt and black pepper to taste

1 cup plain 2% reduced-fat Greek yogurt

2 tablespoons grated onion

1 tablespoon peeled and grated fresh ginger

1 tablespoon olive oil
1 tablespoon ground cumin
1 tablespoon paprika
½ teaspoon ground turmeric
3 cloves garlic, minced

1. Prepare the quinoa according to the package directions, using broth instead of water and adding the garlic powder to the preparation. When done, add in the avocado, spinach, and salt to taste. There is no need for additional cooking; the spinach will wilt from the heat of the quinoa. Cover with a lid and set aside.

2. Make the salmon: Turn on your oven's broiler and set the rack 6 inches away from the heat source. Line a pan with foil (or no foil if you prefer) and apply cooking spray. Place the salmon on the baking sheet and season with salt and pepper to your liking.

3. In a bowl mix together the yogurt, onion, ginger, olive oil, cumin, paprika, turmeric, and garlic.

4. Broil the salmon for 2 to 4 minutes. Remove from the broiler and evenly slather the fillets with the spiced yogurt mixture. Return to the broiler and continue to broil for an additional 3 to 4 minutes. Serve with the quinoa.

A BETTER MAC AND CHEESE

Your gluten- and dairy-sensitive child can still have mac and cheese, thanks to Donna Gordon-Teixeira, who created most of the gluten-free baked goodies for this book. Turn it into a healthy veggie casserole by adding a small handful each of chopped broccoli, mushrooms, spinach, and onions, and placing it in a casserole topped with extra cheese.

Makes 2 to 3 servings

2 cups gluten-free and casein-free macaroni noodles, such as
    Tinkyada
1½ to 2 cups Daiya Cheese Cheddar Shreds

4 tablespoons Earth Balance buttery spread

¼ cup rice or coconut milk, such as So Delicious

¼ teaspoon black pepper

1 teaspoon sea salt

1. Preheat the oven to 350°F.

2. In a Dutch oven or other oven-safe pot, cook the noodles for 16 minutes at a rapid boil. Drain in cold water.

3. In the same pan you used to cook the noodles, add the cheese, butter spread, milk, pepper, and salt and cook over low heat until the cheese begins to melts. Add the noodles back to the pan until the desired thickness is achieved.

4. Bake until golden-brown.

GARBANZO BEAN FRIED CHICKEN

Stacey Gadbois of Virginia Beach, Virginia, and her daughter, Emma, both have food sensitivities, so Stacey has spent years perfecting recipes that would both protect their health and please the entire family. She came up with a healthier version of a kid favorite—Southern fried chicken—by substituting garbanzo bean flour as a gluten-free alternative to white flour. "It adds a rich nutty flavor," she says, "but it needs salt and spices." Her family likes plenty of flavor, so if this is not your style, adjust the seasonings accordingly to suit your family's taste buds. She also recommends using a deep fryer when working with garbanzo flour, as the coating tends to get soggy when pan-fried. If you don't have or can't find garbanzo bean flour, you can use rice flour. Make sure to drain the chicken well before serving.

Makes 4 servings

1 cup garbanzo bean flour or brown rice flour

4 teaspoons sea salt

½ teaspoon onion salt

½ teaspoon garlic salt

1 teaspoon Italian seasoning
1 teaspoon black pepper
2 eggs, beaten, or ½ cup olive oil
Safflower oil for frying
1 pound boneless, skinless chicken breast, sliced into strips

1. Combine the flour, salt, onion salt, garlic salt, Italian seasoning, and pepper in a bowl. Put the beaten eggs or oil in a separate bowl.

2. Dip each chicken strip in the egg mixture or oil, then in the flour mixture. Coat well. Put in deep fryer according to manufacturer's directions and fry until golden and cooked through, 5 to 10 minutes. Drain the chicken on paper towels to remove excess oil before serving.

KIDS LOVE KETCHUP

Stacey Gadbois of Virginia Beach, Virginia, used trial and error to come up with this all-natural ketchup a few years ago when her daughter, Emma, then age 2, loved "dip-dip" but couldn't tolerate the store-bought condiment. She's recently revised it, and her daughter says, "It's better than ever." Most important, it avoids the high-fructose corn syrup found in manufactured ketchup that her daughter could not tolerate. And it only takes 10 minutes to make. Of course, if your child can't tolerate tomatoes, these recipes are not for your family.

STACEY'S ALL-NATURAL
HOMEMADE KETCHUP

Makes about 4 cups

Two 28-ounce cans crushed tomatoes, drained
1 tablespoon tomato paste

½ cup apple cider vinegar

3 tablespoons coconut nectar

½ cup xylitol

1 teaspoon onion powder

½ teaspoon garlic powder

2 teaspoons sea salt

⅛ teaspoon celery salt

⅛ teaspoon mustard powder

¼ teaspoon black pepper

1 whole clove

Using the back of a spatula, strain the crushed tomatoes through a small-holed strainer to remove the seeds. Put the tomatoes with the rest of the ingredients in a large saucepan or stockpot and bring to a simmer over medium-low heat. Cook, stirring occasionally with a whisk, for 1½ hours. Remove the clove and cool. The ketchup will keep in an airtight container in the refrigerator for up to 2 weeks.

STACEY'S CARIBBEAN-STYLE BBQ SAUCE

Add an extra 5 minutes to already quick Stacey's All-Natural Homemade Ketchup and take it with you to the outdoor grill.

Makes about 2 cups

1 cup Stacey's All-Natural Homemade Ketchup (above)

3 tablespoons apple cider vinegar

1 tablespoon coconut oil

1½ tablespoons coconut nectar

½ cup natural, pure maple syrup

1 tablespoon onion powder

½ tablespoon ground mustard
½ teaspoon sea salt
½ teaspoon garlic powder

Place all of the ingredients in a medium saucepan, stir well, and bring to a slow boil. Reduce the heat and simmer, uncovered, for 20 minutes, stirring occasionally. Cool before storing. This sauce will keep in an airtight container in the refrigerator for 2 weeks.

COCONUT-CRUSTED CHICKEN FINGERS[2]

Connie Portman of the Brain Balance Achievement Center in Tulsa, Oklahoma, found this the perfect healthy way to wean children off the chicken fingers they love at fast-food places and other restaurants, which are always breaded and deep-fried. These healthier alternatives are a perfect blend of sweet, crunchy, and savory flavors.

Makes 6 to 8 servings

2 pounds boneless, skinless chicken breast
2 cups almond flour
1½ cups unsweetened shredded coconut
1 teaspoon sea salt
¼ teaspoon black pepper
¼ teaspoon ground ginger
3 large eggs
1 tablespoon water
1 tablespoon agave nectar
2 tablespoons olive oil

1. Preheat the oven to 350°F.

---

2 This recipe contains eggs so do not use it if your child cannot tolerate or is sensitive to eggs.

2. Place the chicken breasts in a 1-gallon Ziploc freezer bag and pound them to ½-inch thickness. Remove them from the bag and cut them into 1-inch strips. Set aside.

3. In a large mixing bowl combine the flour, coconut, salt, pepper, and ginger.

4. In a small bowl whisk together the eggs, water, and agave.

5. Dip each strip in the egg mixture, then roll in the coconut mixture to coat evenly. Place on a baking sheet sprayed with nonstick spray. Bake for 25 minutes, turning once halfway through.

SASSY SALSAS

Next to ketchup, the condiment that just might be a kid's favorite could be salsa. This duo was created by Jordan S. Rubin, NMD, PhD, bestselling author of *The Maker's Diet* and founder of Beyond Organic, a company that specializes in manufacturing nutrient-dense farm-to-consumer foods and other health products.

MANGO-AVOCADO SALSA

Makes about 3 cups

1 ripe avocado, pitted and cut into small cubes
1 ripe mango, pitted and cut into small cubes
½ cup minced red bell pepper
1 jalapeño pepper, seeded and diced
1 tablespoon fresh lime juice
2 tablespoons finely chopped fresh cilantro
1 tablespoon finely chopped fresh parsley
1 teaspoon coconut sugar

Combine all of the ingredients in a medium bowl and stir well. Refrigerate until ready to serve.

CHUNKY TOMATO SALSA

This salsa makes a nice accompaniment to chicken and guacamole.

Makes about 4 cups

3 vine-ripened fresh tomatoes, diced
⅔ cup fresh cilantro
1 diced jalapeño pepper
¼ cup diced red onion
Juice of two fresh limes
Juice of half an orange
Sea salt and black pepper to taste

Mix all of the ingredients in a medium bowl and refrigerate until ready to use.

FRIED CHICKEN TENDERS[3]

Another way to fuel a kid's love of fried chicken comes from Tony T., a Brain Balance dad from Wake Forest, North Carolina. Tony does a lot of the family cooking and perfected this recipe for his chicken tenders–loving son who is sensitive to gluten. "It's hard to come up with recipes that an elementary school student will eat and will be good for him too," says Tony, "but he loves this." You can change the recipe any way you need to address food sensitivities—almond or soy milk instead of cow's milk, canola or coconut oil instead of peanut oil, or even add some herbs of your liking to the batter. If your child can tolerate eggs, you can substitute one beaten large egg for the xanthan gum mixture.

Makes 8 servings

---

3 Eliminate the lemon if your child is sensitive to citrus. Also, corn and corn products are chief suspects as a food sensitivity, so do not use this recipe if you find out your child is allergic to the grain.

FOR THE MARINADE

> 2½ cups milk
>
> Juice of one lemon
>
> 1 to 1½ teaspoons sea salt
>
> 1 teaspoon black pepper
>
> 3 pounds chicken tenders

FOR THE BATTER

> 1 cup gluten-free flour, such as Donna's GF All-Purpose Flour (page 188)
>
> 1½ tablespoons xanthan gum
>
> ¾ cup water
>
> 3 to 4 cups panko-style corn bread crumbs or cornmeal

FOR FRYING

> Enough peanut or coconut oil to fill a deep skillet 3 inches deep

1. Make the marinade: Combine all of the marinade ingredients except the chicken in a gallon Ziploc bag and shake. Add the chicken and make sure all the chicken pieces are well coated. If possible, let the tenders marinate in the refrigerator overnight, turning the bag over once.

2. When you're ready to cook, drain the marinade from the bag and remove the chicken tenders. Discard the marinade. Lightly pat the chicken pieces with paper towel to remove any drippings.

3. To prepare the batter, put the flour on a small plate. In a small bowl, mix the xanthan gum and water and whisk to a thin paste. The xanthan gum tends to tighten up the mixture, so you may need to adjust the amount of water. Start with a little less and add more as needed. Make sure there are no lumps. Put the corn bread crumbs on a large plate.

4. One at a time, take a chicken tender and lightly coat it with the flour. Shake off any excess. You want just enough coating so the xanthan gum mixture will stick to it. Dip the floured tender in the mixture and dredge in the corn bread crumbs. Transfer each piece to a large plate to

await frying. This step will make your hands messy, so you can use tongs, if you prefer.

5. Preheat a wok or deep skillet to medium-high heat. When hot, pour in enough oil to measure about 3 inches. The oil is ready when a few corn kernels placed in the oil fry and pop. Gently place enough tenders in the pan to make one layer, with room between each piece. Fry for 2 minutes. Using tongs, gently turn the tenders and fry for 2 minutes longer. The chicken will become very hard on the outside and golden-brown. Remove to a paper towel–lined plate and continue with the rest of the tenders.

CRISPY PAN-FRIED CHICKEN

The Savvy Gluten-Free Shopper author Jennifer Fugo says it doesn't take fancy ingredients to make moist, crispy chicken, and she proved it when she made this simple recipe during a demonstration and book signing at a Williams-Sonoma store near her suburban Philadelphia home. "People couldn't believe how moist and tender it was," she says, "especially without added fat." Kids will love the crispy texture. The secret, she says, is to not disturb the chicken in the pan so it renders its own fat. "Resist the urge to move it around, even though it will initially be sticky in the pan," she says. If you can't find boneless chicken thighs with the skin intact, buy a regular package of thighs and remove the bone with a paring knife.

Makes 4 servings

4 boneless chicken thighs with skin
Sea salt to taste
Freshly ground black pepper to taste

1. Rinse and pat dry the thighs. Salt them evenly on both sides.

2. Heat a heavy-bottomed skillet over medium heat and add the thighs, skin side down, to the dry pan. Cook, undisturbed, for 15 minutes, or until the fat is rendered and the skin yields when you move the thighs in the pan. Turn the thighs and cook for 5 minutes more, or until cooked through. Sprinkle with pepper and serve.

CHICKEN FOR EVERY DAY, ANY WAY

Lisa Carlson, the director of the Brain Balance Achievement Center in Minnetonka, Minnesota, makes feeding her family easy by cooking up a large batch of chicken on the weekend that she can transform into soups, salads, sandwiches, or casseroles for meals during the week. She uses it to make a quick chicken soup, including her Coconut Curry Soup (page 136), a convenient protein fill for midweek tacos—always a kid favorite—or an easy-to-assemble chicken casserole. On many days she sends her son to school with a chicken-based soup in a thermos to make sure he gets his protein. The easiest thing about this recipe, says Lisa, is that you can add anything you have on hand to the pot to flavor the chicken. It needn't be precise.

LISA'S MULTIPURPOSE CHICKEN

Makes enough for several meals

10 to 12 boneless, skinless chicken breasts
One 32-ounce box low-sodium chicken stock
½ cup chopped onion
1 tablespoon chopped garlic
2 teaspoons herbs de Provence or any combination of
 herbs of choice

Put the chicken breasts in a large skillet or Dutch oven. Add only as much as will fit one layer. You do not want to crowd them. Add the broth and remaining ingredients and bring to a simmer. Cover and simmer until cooked through, about 30 minutes. Remove to a plate to cool. Repeat with the remaining chicken. Store in a container in the refrigerator or freezer for later use.

MOROCCAN CHICKEN SALAD

This is a salad kids actually ask for! "At my house we serve this as a dinner salad and as leftovers over rice the next day," says Rebecca Jackson of the Brain Balance Achievement Center in Midlothian, Virginia, and the centers in Cary and Chapel Hill in North Carolina. With such a variety of vegetables and the aromatic spices, there is plenty of flavor, so there is no need for dressing. If you want a dressing, however, she recommends oil and vinegar or a simple vinaigrette. The salad can be served warm or chilled.

Makes about 10 servings

Coconut-oil cooking spray
2 large or 3 small fresh beets, peeled and sliced
1 butternut squash, peeled and diced
1 cup peeled and diced carrots
4 whole boneless, skinless chicken breasts
1 teaspoon ground cumin
1 teaspoon ground turmeric
1 teaspoon ground nutmeg
1 teaspoon ground cinnamon
1 teaspoon ground coriander
1 tablespoon coconut oil
6 cups mixed baby greens
2 avocados, pitted and diced
½ cup diced dates
½ cup craisins
½ cup slivered almonds

1. Preheat the oven to 350°F.

2. Coat a cookie sheet with coconut-oil cooking spray. Spread the vegetables out on the sheet and roast for 20 to 30 minutes, or until just tender.

3. While the vegetables are roasting, prepare the chicken: Wash and dry the breasts. Mix the spices together in a small bowl and sprinkle them

over both sides of the breasts. Add the coconut oil to a large skillet over medium heat. When melted, add the chicken and sauté for about 10 minutes, or until the chicken is cooked through. Cut into bite-size pieces.

4. Put the greens in the bottom of a large serving bowl. Layer the beets, then the squash and carrots on top. Add the chicken, then the avocados, dates, craisins, and almonds.

TURKEY POTPIE

A perfect old-school comfort food, updated by Brain Balance corporate nutrition director Christie Korth to please picky palates and accommodate food sensitivities. And the bonus? "I think it tastes even better than the original," she says.

Makes 4 to 6 servings

Gluten-free pizza dough for a double-crust pie
½ cup Earth Balance spread
½ cup Donna's GF All-Purpose Flour (page 188) or packaged gluten-free flour
1 teaspoon sea salt
Dash black pepper
¼ cup plus ⅓ cup rice milk, divided
2 cups low-sodium chicken broth
3 cups cooked cubed turkey
1 cup chopped spinach
3 potatoes, cooked, peeled, and cubed
One 16-ounce package frozen mixed vegetables
½ teaspoon dried thyme

1. Preheat the oven to 375°F.

2. Divide the pizza dough in half. Roll out half of the dough on a lightly floured surface into a 14-inch circle. Gently fit into a 2-quart deep-dish round casserole dish. Trim the pastry to 1 inch from edge of the dish. Set aside. Roll out the remaining dough on a lightly floured surface into a second 14-inch circle. Set aside.

3. In medium saucepan melt the Earth Balance spread. Add the flour, salt, and pepper and stir until combined. Slowly add ¼ cup of the rice milk and the chicken broth and cook over medium heat, stirring constantly, until thick and smooth. Remove from the heat and pour into a large bowl. Add the ⅓ cup of rice milk and mix well. Stir in the remaining ingredients. Spoon into the pie crust.

4. Cover the casserole dish with the remaining dough. Fold a 1-inch strip around the top edges of the pastry. Crimp to seal. Cut four slits in the top to vent. Brush the pastry with water. Bake for 60 to 70 minutes, or until golden-brown. Let stand 10 minutes before serving.

BEST STORE-BOUGHT SUBSTITUTIONS

Hands down, our Brain Balance Achievement Centers recommend these brands as substitutions for certain food sensitivities:

Dairy-free beverages to desserts: So Delicious offers a huge line of really tasty casein-free products, ranging from milks, creamers, and yogurts to frozen desserts. It was a top casein-free choice of recipe developers.

Cheese: Daiya brand is dairy free and soy free and comes sliced or shredded in Cheddar and mozzarella. Daiya also makes a cream cheese substitute. It is another top choice of our recipe developers.

Butter: Earth Balance makes a variety of spreads that are both dairy free and soy free. Our recipes developers loved this product for the way it worked in recipes.

Cream: Whole Foods's 365 Everyday Value brand canned Organic Coconut Milk. Refrigerate the can, which will separate the solid (cream) from the liquid. Skim the cream off the top and use it as a thickener for anything that calls for cream. For sour cream, add a little lemon to the "cream" and thin it with rice milk.

Gluten-free sandwich bread and bagels: Udi's brand.

Nutrition bars: Caveman brand bars are all natural, gluten-free, and contain no peanuts. Also, LäraBars, Kind (with and without peanuts), and Van's.

Flour: Namaste Foods Gluten-Free Perfect Flour Blend, which already includes xanthan gum.

Many of these brands can be found in markets that cater to customers on gluten-free diets.

TURKEY, CABBAGE, AND CARROTS OVER RICE

If your family likes Chinese food, this dish is a family-pleasing healthier tradeoff that accommodates most all food sensitivities, says Stacey Gadbois.

Makes 4 to 6 servings

3 tablespoons olive oil
1 large yellow onion, diced
1 head green cabbage, chopped into small pieces
6 carrots, peeled and chopped
Sea salt and black pepper to taste
2 pounds ground turkey
2 to 3 cups hot cooked brown rice

1. Heat 2 tablespoons of the olive oil in a large skillet over medium heat. Add the onion and sauté for 5 minutes. Add the cabbage, carrots, and salt and pepper to taste. Lower the heat, cover, and continue to cook for 20 to 30 minutes, or until the cabbage and carrots are soft.

2. In a separate skillet, brown the ground turkey in the remaining tablespoon of olive oil until cooked through, about 8 minutes.

3. To serve, divide the rice among 4 to 6 dinner plates. Spoon turkey over the rice and top with the vegetable mixture.

SLOW-COOKER PORK CHOPS

The Brain Balance Achievement Center in Tulsa, Oklahoma, offers this slow-cooker recipe for busy parents. Team it up with mashed potatoes and a green salad.

Makes 4 servings

2 tablespoons olive oil
4 boneless pork chops, each about ½-inch thick
1 cup chicken broth
2 cloves garlic, minced
1 teaspoon dried oregano
½ teaspoon black pepper
¼ teaspoon sea salt

1. Heat 1 tablespoon of the olive oil in a sauté pan. Add the pork chops and cook over medium-high heat to sear and lightly brown, about 3 minutes on each side.

2. Place the chops in the bottom of a slow cooker. It's okay to layer them. Add the broth and sprinkle with the garlic, oregano, pepper, and salt. Drizzle the remaining olive oil over the top. Cover and cook on low for 4 to 6 hours, or until the chops are cooked through.

GARBANZO BEAN FRIED SHRIMP

Kids love fried shrimp! This version, developed by Stacey Gadbois, uses gluten-free garbanzo bean flour instead of white flour, and safflower oil for the deep-frying. **Note:** You can cut back by half on the salt and garlic powder for a milder flavor.

Makes 4 servings

1 cup garbanzo bean flour or brown rice flour
4 teaspoons sea salt
2 teaspoons garlic powder
2 teaspoons onion salt
1 teaspoon black pepper
2 eggs, beaten, or ½ cup olive oil

1 pound shrimp, shelled and deveined

Safflower oil for deep-frying

1. Combine the flour, salt, garlic powder, onion salt, and pepper in a bowl. Put the beaten eggs or oil in a separate bowl.

2. Dip each shrimp in the egg mixture, then the flour mixture. Coat well. Put in deep fryer according to manufacturer's directions and fry until golden and cooked through, 3 to 5 minutes. Drain on paper towels.

LINGUINE ALFREDO

Alfredo without dairy, eggs, or cheese? You got it! It's tough to deprive a pasta- and cheese-loving child of a dish she loves to eat. Now you don't have to, thanks to Hadley McGregor of the Brain Balance Achievement Center in Huntington Beach, California.

Makes 4 servings

8 ounces (half a box) gluten-free rice pasta

¼ cup rice milk

½ cup Smart Balance soy-free margarine

1 cup Daiya mozzarella-flavored cheese

¼ teaspoon garlic powder

¼ teaspoon onion powder

¼ teaspoon ground black pepper

½ cup chopped fresh parsley

1. Bring 4 quarts of water and a teaspoon of salt to a boil in a medium to large pot. (Add a drop of oil to prevent the pasta from sticking). Add the pasta and boil according to the package directions (5 to 7 minutes). Drain the pasta and rinse with cold water.

2. Return the rinsed pasta to the empty pot and add the rice milk. Bring to a low boil. Gradually mix in the margarine, cheese, garlic powder, onion powder, and pepper until the sauce has a creamy consistency. Add the parsley for garnish and serve.

GRUB WORMS AND DIRT BOMBS[4]

Here's a new take on spaghetti and meatballs. "After working for years with children who are picky eaters, I have found one of the best ways to get them to eat their fruits and veggies is to make them fun, entertaining, and appealing to the eyes," says Brain Balance corporate nutrition director Christie Korth. "The 'worms' in this dish are the noodles, and the rest looks like a blob of earth. Kids love the presentation."

Makes 6 servings

1½ pounds ground turkey
¼ small red bell pepper, diced
2 cloves garlic, diced
2 scallions, finely chopped
1 teaspoon grated fresh ginger
2 tablespoons barbecue sauce, such as Stacey's Caribbean-Style BBQ Sauce (page 144)
1 teaspoon sea salt
3 tablespoons olive oil
1 cup shredded carrots
1 cup bean sprouts
1 cup snow peas
1 pound cooked Asian wide rice noodles, made according to package directions
¼ cup gluten-free tamari

1. Preheat the oven to 350°F.

2. In a mixing bowl combine the ground turkey, red bell pepper, garlic, scallions, ginger, barbecue sauce, and salt. Roll meatball-like into small "dirt bombs," which should give you about two dozen. Place the dirt bombs on a nonstick cooking sheet coated lightly with nonstick spray. Bake for 10 to 12 minutes.

---

4 Do not serve this recipe if you determine that your child is sensitive to tomatoes (and therefore BBQ sauce).

3. Meanwhile, heat the oil in a large skillet and add the carrots, bean sprouts, and snow peas. Cook for 5 minutes. Add the cooked noodles and tamari; combine, and heat through. Remove the turkey meatballs from the oven and serve with the pasta.

SPAGHETTI AND SPANISH MEATBALLS

Pork meatballs are a family favorite in Stacey Gadbois's household. "This recipe is just aromatic enough to add some Mediterranean flare," says Stacey, who has to adjust family meals to accommodate her own and her daughter's food sensitivities. If you don't prefer the heat, as her family does, omit the red pepper.

Makes 4 servings

1 pound ground pork
3 cloves garlic, pressed
1 teaspoon coriander or 1 tablespoon diced cilantro
¼ to ½ teaspoon diced hot red pepper (optional)
Sea salt and black pepper to taste
3 cups cooked brown rice pasta

1. Preheat the oven to 350°F.

2. Combine all of the ingredients, except the pasta, in a mixing bowl. Shape into 2- to 3-inch-round meatballs. Spray a baking dish with nonstick spray and bake for 20 minutes, or until cooked through and no longer pink inside. Serve with the pasta.

STUFFED ACORN SQUASH

This is a fall favorite in Rebecca Jackson's household. "Kids love using the squash as a bowl," she says, "and adding the craisins helps to sweeten the dish and make the taste more appealing."

Makes 6 servings

3 acorn squash
1 cup raw quinoa
2 tablespoons grapeseed or coconut oil

1 medium onion, chopped
3 stalks celery, minced
1 tablespoon minced garlic
3 whole chicken breasts, diced
1 cup sliced mushrooms
½ cup craisins
¼ teaspoon ground cinnamon

1. Preheat the oven to 350°F.

2. Cut the squash in half and scoop out the seeds. Place in a baking pan with the "cup" end up. Pour ¼ cup of water around the squash and bake for 1 hour. Remove from the oven.

3. While the squash is cooking, prepare the quinoa according to the package directions.

4. Heat the oil in a large skillet over medium heat. Add the onion, celery, and garlic and sauté until soft, about 3 minutes. Add the chicken and mushrooms and continue to sauté until the chicken is cooked through, 5 to 10 minutes.

5. Combine the cooked quinoa and chicken mixture in a large bowl and stir together.

6. Remove the squash from the oven and, using a fork, lightly scrape the sides to loosen some of the squash. Using the baked squash as a bowl, add the chicken-and-quinoa mixture. Sprinkle with the craisins and cinnamon and serve.

STUFFED RED BELL PEPPERS

The mushrooms and beef add a richness to the sweet tang of the red pepper—a great combo, courtesy of Stacey Gadbois.

Makes 4 servings

¼ cup olive oil
1½ pounds lean ground beef
1¼ cups sliced fresh mushrooms, such as button, portabella, or shiitake

½ white onion, diced
1 teaspoon garlic salt
Sea salt and black pepper to taste
2 quarts water
4 small red bell peppers, halved and seeded

1. Preheat the oven to 375°F.

2. Heat the olive oil in a large skillet over medium heat. Add the ground beef and brown, stirring frequently. Halfway through browning, add the mushrooms and onion. Continue cooking until the meat is cooked through. Season with the garlic salt and salt and pepper and set aside.

3. Meanwhile, bring the water to a boil in a medium saucepan. Using tongs, gently place the bell pepper halves in the water and boil for 2 minutes. You can do this a few at a time. Remove the peppers and place them, hollow side up, in a 9 x 13-inch baking dish. Divide the beef mixture equally among the peppers. Bake for 20 minutes.

DR. DAVE'S MOLÉ CHILI[5]

My friend and colleague Dr. David A. Gentile uses neutraceuticals and a culinary approach to health and healing at his Oasis Integrative Medicine practice in Rocky Point, New York. He's even developed his own recipes featuring foods, spices, and herbs that have been found to promote health and healing in a variety of ways. Here's one of them. How are your kids going to resist a chili recipe made with real chocolate! "Adjust the ingredients to your own taste," he says. "Have fun with your creativity." Garnish with any of these flavors to taste: chopped scallions, sliced avocado, low-fat sour cream, chopped chilies, and cilantro. Serve over rice or with fresh corn tortillas.

Makes 8 to 10 servings

---

5   Do not use this recipe if your child is sensitive to beans or corn.

2 tablespoons olive oil

2 medium onions, diced

6 cloves garlic, diced

2 pounds lean free-range ground beef

One 16-ounce can red kidney beans, drained and rinsed

One 15-ounce can fire-roasted crushed tomatoes

1 teaspoon ground cumin

1 teaspoon chili powder

1 teaspoon ground cinnamon

1 teaspoon chipotle pepper

Sea salt and black pepper to taste

6 ounces 87 to 93 percent dark chocolate, crumbled

1. Heat the olive oil over medium heat in a large deep skillet or Dutch oven. Add the onions and garlic and sauté until soft. Add the ground beef and sauté until browned.

2. Add the beans, tomatoes, cumin, chili powder, cinnamon, chipotle, and salt and pepper to taste. Stir and cook for 10 minutes.

3. Stir in the chocolate until it melts, bring to a simmer, cover, and cook for 2 hours. If the chili gets too thick, add some beef broth to thin it out.

SWEET POTATO/BLACK BEAN BURRITOS IN COLLARD WRAPS[6]

This twist on the traditional bean burrito substitutes super-nutritious collard greens for the tortillas. And, with the addition of sweet potatoes, it makes for one healthy dish. Kristen Davidson, nutrition coach of the Brain Balance Achievement Center in Overland Park, Kansas, says it's easy to be creative when building these burritos with other add-ins, such as diced avocado, salsa, or cashew cheese for the dairy sensitive.

Makes 4 servings

---

6   Do not make this recipe if your child is sensitive to beans. If your child is sensitive to lime, eliminate it from the recipe.

2 pounds sweet potatoes, peeled and chopped into
   ¾-inch pieces
1 onion, diced
1 green bell pepper, diced
2 cloves garlic, diced
3 tablespoons melted coconut oil
1 pound grass-fed ground beef
2 teaspoons chili powder
1 teaspoon ground cumin
1 teaspoon ground coriander
Sea salt to taste
Juice of 1 lime
½ cup chopped tomatoes
2½ cups canned black beans, drained and rinsed
¼ cup chopped cilantro
8 large collard leaves

1. Preheat the oven to 400°F.

2. Put the sweet potato, onion, bell pepper, and garlic in a mixing bowl. Add 2 tablespoons of the coconut oil and toss. Make sure the vegetables are well coated. Transfer to a baking pan and roast for 40 minutes.

3. Meanwhile, sauté the ground beef over medium heat with the remaining coconut oil in a large frying pan. Add the chili powder, cumin, coriander, and salt and continue cooking until the beef is cooked through, about 10 minutes.

4. Add the lime juice, tomatoes, beans, and roasted vegetables to the beef. Combine well. Add the cilantro and adjust the seasonings to taste.

5. Lay out the collard leaves. Divide the mixture down the center of each leaf, and fold up like a burrito.

SPICING IT UP

Mexican and Southwestern food would not be the same without the spiciness that comes from a seasoning blend. The only thing is, it's almost impossible to find a prepackaged version that doesn't contain something that many Brain Balance kids are sensitive to. Beth V., a mother at the Brain Balance Achievement Center in Edwardsville, Illinois, comes to the rescue with this taco mix that is free of gluten, soy, egg, and dairy. And it's so easy to mix up a batch—just takes a few minutes. The recipe is enough to mix into 2 pounds of ground meat.

TACO SEASONING

Makes about ½ cup

1 tablespoon chili powder
1½ teaspoons ground cumin
1 teaspoon sea salt
1 teaspoon black pepper
½ teaspoon paprika
¼ teaspoon garlic powder
¼ teaspoon onion powder
¼ teaspoon crushed red pepper flakes
¼ teaspoon dried oregano

Grind all the ingredients in an electric spice grinder or mini food processor. If you don't have either appliance, just combine them well in a bowl. Use right away or store in a small glass container until ready to use.

Chapter 9
More Vegetables and Fruit, Please!

These are words seldom heard from the mouths of babes, but it *can* happen. One strategy is full family participation. As I said in Chapter 4, *you* have to be the role model. *You* have to make the effort. Getting your kids to eat more fruits and vegetables is really up to you.

People in the United States consume far fewer fruits and vegetables than in any other country in the world. That's pretty sad when you consider that most of us have access to just about anything we want and fresh, organic fruits and vegetables are readily available in many supermarkets these days. Vegetables should be at the top of the list for every meal you plan. *All* kids could stand to eat more vegetables.

The number-one thing missing from the typical kid's diet is leafy greens, like Swiss chard, collards, romaine, bok choy, and arugula. They all contain copious amounts of vitamin A, D, E, and K in addition to important minerals, including calcium, magnesium, and iron.

The easiest way to get more vegetables in the diet is to add them to soup, especially if your children don't like salads. When cooked, greens lose their bitterness. I know one mom who puts pureed spinach in her tomato sauce, though her kids will tell everyone they hate spinach. Sometimes you just have to be a little creative. You also do not need to shop every day. If fresh vegetables are not available or if they are too expensive for your budget, fill your freezer with frozen vegetables and serve them at every meal. Frozen vegetables are just as nutritious as fresh because they are usually flash frozen when picked. On special occasions, or when you feel like getting a little fancy, try one of the following recipes. We know kids really go for them.

CAJUN RED POTATO FRIES

Rusty Hamlin, the popular executive chef for Zac Brown Band's Eat and Greets, has personal experience in how to lure kids into trying new foods. Starting when he was four years old, his mother would sit him on the kitchen counter while she was preparing dinner and have him sample what was on the menu. Rusty got a nickel for every taste nuance he could identify. The experience inspired him to pursue a profession in the culinary arts. Today, Brain Balance kids are discovering that his Cajun oven-baked fries are a great substitute for French fries.

Makes 6 to 8 servings

12 medium red potatoes
3 tablespoons olive oil
3 tablespoons Cajun seasoning
3 tablespoons chopped fresh parsley
2 tablespoons granulated garlic

1. Preheat the oven to 375°F.

2. Cut the potatoes in wedges, about six per potato. Put the oil, seasoning, parsley, and garlic in a large mixing bowl and toss in the potato wedges. Stir to cover completely and evenly.

3. Place the potatoes on a greased baking pan and roast for 40 minutes, or until crisp.

JOSH PRICHARD'S KICKIN' VEGAN POTATO SALAD

Josh Prichard is a chef who travels with the Zac Brown Band to prepare food for his Eat and Greet concerts. This potato salad is a hit with the fans. You can use the same dressing with cabbage and carrots to fix a yummy slaw.

Makes 8 servings

FOR THE DRESSING

1 cup Veganaise
1 tablespoon kosher salt, plus more to taste
1 tablespoon garlic powder
1 tablespoon agave nectar
3 tablespoons creole mustard
1 lime, zested and juiced
¼ cup coconut vinegar
1 tablespoon sriracha (or more or less depending on preferred heat)
Freshly ground black pepper to taste

FOR THE POTATOES

3½ pounds baby red potatoes
1½ gallons water
3 tablespoons sea salt
1 large sweet onion, diced fine
6 stalks celery, finely diced
¼ cup chives, chopped fine

1. To make the dressing: In a medium bowl whisk together all of the dressing ingredients. Refrigerate until ready to use.

2. To prepare the potatoes: Put the potatoes in a medium stockpot with the water and salt. Bring the potatoes to a boil on high heat, reduce to a simmer, and cook until tender, about 20 minutes. Drain and cool. Chop the potatoes to a medium dice.

3. In a large mixing bowl combine the cooked potatoes, diced vegetables, chives, and dressing and lightly toss. Refrigerate until ready to eat.

CINNAMON-SPICED SWEET POTATOES

Sweet potatoes are a super-healthy food rich in antioxidants, so you want to make sure to include them in your family's diet. "We didn't want to miss having candied sweet potatoes of some sort at Thanksgiving, so I came up with this xylitol-sweetened version," says Stacey Gadbois, who helps show parents at the Brain Balance

Achievement Center in Virginia Beach, Virginia, how to adjust their cooking for kids with food sensitivities. Coconut oil is a healthy alternative to butter and also gives this dish an extra kick.

Makes 4 servings

> 2 large sweet potatoes in their jackets
> ¾ cup coconut oil
> ¼ cup xylitol
> 1 to 2 tablespoons ground cinnamon

1. Preheat the oven to 350°F.

2. Wash the sweet potatoes and cut them into ½-inch slices. Spray a 9 x 13-inch baking dish with nonstick spray. Put the sweet potato slices in the dish in a single layer, overlapping slightly. Drizzle with the coconut oil. Top with the xylitol and cinnamon and bake for 25 to 30 minutes, or until soft.

SWEET POTATO FRIES

French fries could possibly be a little kid's favorite food, and the children at the Brain Balance Achievement Center in Bluffton, South Carolina, give this slight twist high fives, says Heather Lowenthal, director. They like the bite they get from the added spices.

Makes 3 to 4 servings

> 1 medium to large sweet potato with skin
> 1 tablespoon olive oil
> 1 teaspoon ground nutmeg
> 1 teaspoon garlic powder
> 1 teaspoon sea salt
> Pinch ground cloves

1. Preheat the oven to 350°F.

2. Wash and pat dry the sweet potato. Cut it into wedges, slices, or strings and put in a mixing bowl. Add the olive oil and seasonings and blend well, making sure all the slices are evenly coated.

3. Put the slices in a single layer in a nonstick baking dish or baking pan. Bake for 30 to 40 minutes, or until the potatoes are light brown along the edges.

GOLDEN BEET SALAD WITH RAINBOW CARROTS, CUCUMBER, AND NUTTY HERB VINAIGRETTE[1]

Rusty Hamlin loves feeding kids almost as much as he does Zac's fans. He designed this recipe to pique their curiosity about carrots—really, they're not always orange?! Rainbow carrots come in a colorful variety from white to purple. If you can't find them, just use regular carrots. If you can't find golden beets, you can use red beets, but you will need to wash them after they are cooked.

Makes 6 servings

FOR THE SALAD
    12 medium-size golden beets
    8 rainbow carrots
    1 seedless cucumber
    1 small red onion, julienned
    1 bunch arugula

FOR THE VINAIGRETTE
    ¼ cup toasted pistachios
    3 cloves garlic
    6 basil leaves
    5 sprigs fresh thyme
    ¼ bunch Italian parsley
    Juice of 3 lemons
    ¼ cup red wine vinegar
    ½ cup olive oil
    Sea salt and black pepper to taste

---

1 Due to the lemon in the dressing, avoid this recipe if you find that your child is sensitive to citrus.

1. To make the salad: Boil the beets in salted water until a toothpick can slide through easily, about 10 minutes. Put the beets in an ice-water bath to cool.

2. When the beets are cool, they will be easy to peel, and the skins should slide off in your hand. Cut the beets in half and slice into thin half-moons.

3. Peel the carrots and slice them into thin rounds. Cut the cucumbers lengthwise, then slice the halves into half-moon slices. Tear the arugula leaves into small pieces. Assemble the vegetables, including the red onion, in a salad bowl.

4. To make the vinaigrette: Place the pistachios and garlic in a blender and pulse a few times to break them down. Add the basil, thyme, parsley, lemon juice, and vinegar and pulse for 20 seconds. Add the olive oil in a slow stream, and continue to blend for 15 seconds. Season to taste.

5. Pour the vinaigrette over the salad and toss.

SOUTH-OF-THE-BORDER SALAD[2]

Friend and colleague Dr. David A. Gentile, known affectionately to his patients at Oasis Integrative Medicine in Rocky Point, New York, as Dr. Dave, loves to share recipes with them. Here's one.

Makes 4 servings

1 pound mixed baby greens
½ cup canned red kidney beans, rinsed
¼ cup chopped red bell pepper
¼ cup chopped green bell pepper
¼ cup chopped fresh tomatoes
¼ cup chopped jícama

Combine all of the ingredients in a large bowl. Dress lightly with your favorite vinaigrette, if desired, and serve.

---

2 Do not make this recipe if you find your child is sensitive to beans or tomatoes.

CRANBERRY CONFETTI WILD RICE

Color overtakes bland-looking rice in this kid-pleasing version from Chef Rusty Hamlin.

Makes 6 servings

1 tablespoon olive oil
1 large onion, chopped
2 large carrots, peeled and diced
2 stalks celery, sliced
2 cloves garlic, minced
3½ cups vegetable broth
½ cup uncooked wild rice
1 cup uncooked long-grain white rice
1 cup dried cranberries
2 tablespoons chopped fresh parsley

1. Heat the oil in a large nonstick pot over medium heat. Add the onion, carrots, celery, and garlic and cook until tender, about 5 minutes. Stir in the broth and wild rice and bring to a boil. Cover and cook over low heat for 25 minutes.

2. Stir in the white rice and dried cranberries. Cover and cook over low heat for 20 minutes, or until the rice is done. Stir in the parsley.

POCKETKNIFE COLESLAW[3]

Kids may turn up their noses at the thought of cabbage, but "stinky cabbage" isn't what comes to mind when you offer Zac Brown's idea of crunchy-sweet coleslaw. Zac's version gets an added kick from horseradish. To make it true Zac-style, you need to use the South's beloved Duke's mayonnaise, but any kind will do.

Makes about 12 servings

---

3 Omit the tomato or avoid this recipe if you find that your child has a sensitivity to it.

1 head green cabbage, about 3 pounds, cored
1 large green bell pepper
2 medium summer-fresh tomatoes
8 scallions, green parts only, sliced ¼-inch thick
2 cups Duke's mayonnaise or other mayonnaise
⅓ cup white vinegar
2 tablespoons horseradish
2 tablespoons yellow mustard
1 tablespoon sugar
1 teaspoon sea salt
½ teaspoon cayenne
½ teaspoon black pepper

1. Cut the cabbage, green pepper, and tomatoes into ¼-inch dice and put in a large mixing bowl.

2. Combine the rest of the ingredients in a medium bowl and mix well. Fold half of the dressing into the vegetables and toss. Add more dressing until you achieve the desired consistency.

TOASTED QUINOA CRAN-RAISIN SALAD

Make your family cookout extra nutritious with this tasty salad. Brain Balance corporate nutrition director Christie Korth, who developed this dish, suggests serving it with grilled salmon or chicken and grilled asparagus.

Makes 4 servings

1 cup quinoa, rinsed well
1¾ cups filtered water or low-sodium chicken broth
¼ cup pine nuts
2 tablespoons extra-virgin olive oil
2 cloves garlic, thinly sliced
⅓ cup chopped fresh parsley
¼ cup raisins
¼ cup dried cranberries
1 tablespoon fresh lemon juice
Sea salt and freshly ground black pepper

1. Put the quinoa in a large saucepan and cook over medium-high heat until toasted, about 2 minutes. Add the water or chicken broth and bring to a boil. Reduce the heat to medium-low and simmer, covered, until the liquid is absorbed, 10 to 15 minutes. Remove from the heat and let sit, covered, for about 2 minutes.

2. Meanwhile, toast the pine nuts in a dry skillet over medium-high heat, stirring, until golden, about 3 minutes; transfer to a plate. Add the olive oil and garlic to the skillet and cook over medium heat, stirring, until golden, about 2 minutes. Transfer the garlic to the plate, reserving the oil.

3. Fluff the quinoa with a fork. Add the pine nuts, garlic, reserved oil, parsley, raisins, cranberries, and lemon juice. Season with salt and pepper and toss for extra flavor.

GRILLED VEGGIE SALAD

The best way to get your kids to eat more salads is to make them irresistible. Gluten Free School founder Jennifer Fugo's secret is to grill vegetables that might not be one of your family's favorites. This salad's colorful display adds to its appeal. It can be prepared on an outdoor or indoor grill.

Makes 4 servings

2 zucchini, sliced lengthwise into ½-inch slices
2 yellow squash, sliced lengthwise into ½-inch slices
2 red bell peppers, tops and seeds removed, quartered
1 pound green beans, trimmed and snapped in half
4 tablespoons olive oil, plus extra for grilling
1 tablespoon red wine vinegar
½ teaspoon sea salt
White pepper to taste

1. Oil the grilling rack and preheat the grill to high, then reduce to medium. Put the zucchini, squash, and peppers in a bowl, add 2 tablespoons of the olive oil, and coat well.

2. Put the green beans in the basket of a steamer and steam over hot water for 3 minutes. Remove to a salad bowl and cover to keep warm.

3. Put the grilling vegetables on the grill until you see grill marks appear, about 3 minutes. When the vegetables start to soften, turn them and brush them with extra oil, if necessary. As the veggies finish, cut them into smaller (1-inch) pieces on a cutting bowl. Add them to the salad bowl.

4. Sprinkle the vegetables with the remaining olive oil, the red wine vinegar, salt, and pepper.

SUMMER FESTIVAL SALAD[4]

Zac Brown's on-the-road chef Rusty Hamlin offers this summer salad, which can be eaten as a main dish, lunch, or dinner side.

Makes 4 servings

FOR THE SALAD

    6 ounces button mushrooms, sliced
    1 medium cucumber, diced
    4 ounces sugar snap peas, trimmed and cut on an angle
    10 ounces cherry tomatoes, halved
    1 small red onion, thinly sliced
    8 ounces fresh mozzarella
    1 ounce fresh (about 20 leaves) basil, roughly chopped
    6 cups mixed greens

FOR THE DRESSING

    ¾ ounce fresh basil (about 12 leaves)
    2 cloves garlic, peeled
    6 ounces fresh raspberries
    ⅓ cup rice vinegar
    ¼ cup extra-virgin olive oil
    2 teaspoons freshly ground black pepper
    1 teaspoon blue agave nectar

1. To make the salad: Combine all of the vegetables except for the greens in a large mixing bowl and set aside.

---

4 Omit the tomatoes if you find that your child is sensitive to them.

2. To make the dressing: Put the basil and garlic in a food processor or blender and blend. Add the raspberries and blend until smooth. Add the remaining ingredients and pulse a few times.

3. Pour three-quarters of the dressing over the vegetables and marinate in the refrigerator for an hour. Reserve the remaining dressing.

4. Divide the greens among four plates. Drizzle with the remaining dressing. Divide the marinated vegetables on top of the greens.

CUCUMBER SALAD

If your child loves cucumbers, take advantage of this souped-up salad, which introduces healthy red bell peppers and purple cabbage into the diet, courtesy of Rusty Hamlin.

Makes 6 servings

2 seedless cucumbers
1 small red onion
1 red bell pepper
½ purple cabbage
¼ cup olive oil
1 tablespoon agave nectar
2 tablespoons chopped fresh dill
1 tablespoon sea salt

1. Slice the cucumbers lengthwise, then slice the halves into thin half-moon-shaped slices. Slice the onion, red bell pepper, and cabbage as thin as possible.

2. Put the olive oil, agave, dill, and salt in a large mixing bowl and whisk to blend. Add the vegetables and toss well to coat. Refrigerate for about 1 hour, tossing the salad every 15 minutes. You can make this salad several hours in advance.

AUTUMN BEAUTY FRUIT SALAD

What a kid-friendly beauty this is! This salad, courtesy of Janeil Swarthout, executive director of the Brain Balance Achievement

Center of Fresno in Clovis, California, is perfect to serve around holiday time, as fresh pomegranates can be found in the market from late October through January.

Makes 6 to 8 servings

6 kiwis, peeled and sliced into rounds
5 persimmons, peeled and sliced
Seeds of ½ pomegranate

Arrange the kiwi and persimmon slices, alternating the colors, on a dish and sprinkle the pomegranate seeds over them.

HAWAIIAN FRUIT SALAD

Anytime you're having a large gathering, try this nutritious tropical fruit salad. "It's always a hit with kids," says Christie Korth. "With all the fruity sweetness, they won't balk about the greens." Another added bonus, Christie says, is that you can start teaching children to eat from all of the colors of the rainbow, as each color denotes a specific health-promoting factor. For example: Feeling blue? The antioxidants in blueberries can actually help increase serotonin and decrease depression.

Makes 10 to 12 servings

FOR THE VINAIGRETTE
½ cup pineapple juice
¼ cup apple cider vinegar
1 shallot, minced
1 clove garlic, minced
Sea salt and black pepper to taste
1 cup coconut oil

FOR THE FRUIT SALAD
1 mango, peeled, pitted, and cut into ¼-inch strips
1 papaya, peeled, seeded, and cut into ¼-inch strips

½ cup raspberries
½ cup sliced bananas
½ cup blueberries
3 golden kiwifruit, peeled and sliced
½ cup chopped macadamia nuts
6 cups spring mix, loosely packed

1. To make the dressing: Whisk together the pineapple juice, cider vinegar, shallot, garlic, and salt and pepper. Slowly incorporate the coconut oil. Set the dressing aside.

2. To make the salad: Toss together the mango, papaya, raspberries, bananas, blueberries, kiwifruit, and macadamia nuts in a salad bowl. Pour in 1 cup of the vinaigrette and blend.

3. Place the spring mix on a large serving tray and top with the mixed fruit.

4. Drizzle the salad with the extra dressing or serve on the side, if desired.

CANDY-CANE CARROTS

What kid would turn down a helping of vegetables with this name! It's the perfect holiday side. Thank you Rusty Hamlin for this creative dish.

Makes 4 servings

¼ cup ground candy canes (reserve ½ tablespoon for garnish)
¼ cup orange marmalade
¼ cup cane syrup
¼ cup rice vinegar
1 tablespoon molasses
1 teaspoon sriracha
1½ pounds carrots, peeled and cut on the bias
½ red onion, julienned
3 ounces dried cherries
3 ounces arugula

1. Preheat the oven to 450°F.

2. Combine 3½ tablespoons of the ground candy canes, the marmalade, cane syrup, rice vinegar, molasses, and sriracha in a small bowl and mix well. Pour the mixture into a high-temperature sauté pan, bring to a simmer, and reduce for 1 minute. Remove from the heat.

3. Add the carrots, red onion, and cherries to the sauté pan and toss well. Transfer to a baking pan. Roast in the oven for 10 minutes, or until glazed. Remove from the oven and toss with the arugula. Garnish with a dusting of ground candy cane.

GREEN BEANS WITH HONEY

If you can't get your kids to eat green beans, try this. Linda Anderson of the Brain Balance Achievement Center of Overland Park (Greater Kansas City) says it's foolproof.

Makes 3 to 4 servings

One 14.5-ounce can green beans
1 tablespoon diced onion or 1 teaspoon dried onion
1 tablespoon honey
Sea salt and black pepper to taste

Put the beans and onion in a medium saucepan over medium heat. Drizzle with the honey and add salt and pepper to taste. Bring to a simmer.

GRILLED ASPARAGUS

Increase your chances of getting your child to eat this nutritious green by making it on the grill, says Chef Rusty Hamlin.

Makes 6 to 8 servings

2 bunches fat asparagus, about 24 stalks
3 tablespoons olive oil
3 tablespoons balsamic vinegar
Sea salt and cracked black pepper to taste

1. Preheat an outdoor grill.

2. Cut off the ends of the asparagus stalks about an inch from the bottom. Put the olive oil, vinegar, and seasonings in a large shallow bowl. Add the asparagus and roll to cover the stalks.

3. Grill the asparagus over medium heat for 10 minutes. Roll the spears around frequently so they cook evenly and get crunchy.

RICE STUFFING

A holiday dinner wouldn't be the same without stuffing, but that's a tall order when you're on a gluten-free diet and can't have bread. This recipe, courtesy of Connie Portman of the Brain Balance Achievement Center in Tulsa, Oklahoma, will allow you to keep tradition going. It offers plenty of protein, fiber, and flavor for a perfect holiday side dish.

Makes 12 servings

3 tablespoons olive oil
1 small onion, diced
1 cup small button mushrooms, sliced
2 cups cooked hot basmati rice
1 cup cooked hot wild rice
¼ cup minced fresh sage leaves
2 tablespoon minced fresh rosemary leaves
2 teaspoons sea salt
½ teaspoon black pepper

Heat the olive oil over medium heat in a medium skillet and sauté the onion and mushrooms until soft. Transfer to a large mixing bowl. Add the rice, sage, rosemary, salt, and pepper and mix well. Serve immediately.

Chapter 10
No-Gluten Baking Your Whole Family Will Love

Birthday cakes, cookies, desserts, Halloween treats. It's heart-wrenching for a parent to deprive their children of these delights just because they can't have gluten. And even though there are gluten-free flours available, making *tasty* foods with them is hardly a slam-dunk.

Nobody knows this better than Donna Gordon-Teixeira, who is legendary for knowing how to bake delicious gluten-free *anything*. I first heard about Donna several years ago when I was in Southern California doing a book signing at Generation Rescue, a national autism organization that provides medical treatment grants to families affected by autism, where Donna is an active volunteer. At the time she also ran the highly acclaimed Art Café and Bakery in San Luis Obispo, which gained notoriety for being on Oprah Winfrey's "favorite things" list. (Sadly, it is now closed.) It had the yummiest selection of gluten-free bread, cookies, muffins, cakes, and other items that you ever tasted. Donna's gluten-free goods became so popular she had to take the business online to keep up with the demand.

Donna's passion to take gluten-free to a higher level was a tribute to a beloved aunt who had died years earlier from complications from undiagnosed celiac disease. It took years of trial and error and lots of mistakes to get her gluten-free goods to the level of what her fans describe as "perfection." She has graciously agreed to share some of what she's learned and, best of all, some of her best recipes with the readers of this book.

If you have a child with a gluten sensitivity, you probably already know what a challenge it is trying to work with gluten-free flours. The elasticity that you're so accustomed to when working with regular dough is not there. "Wheat flour is very predictable and consistent because it has starch and it will have a uniform color," says Donna, "but gluten-free flours will behave differently. You will need to add a starch such as potato, cornstarch, tapioca, or arrowroot every time and, depending on the type of flour you use, you can expect a change in the taste and texture of the recipe."

"Without gluten, you lose elasticity, so adding xanthan or guar gum, which mimic many of the properties of gluten, helps so you don't end up with a brick," says Donna. It improves the texture and allows the dough to stretch, which is very important. The secret to better gluten-free baking is to use a mixture of flours rather than just one type, she says. You should also use different mixtures for different types of baked goods. Darker flours, such as whole-grain brown rice flour, millet flour, sorghum flour, and cornmeal flour, are better for items such as pizza crusts, cornbread tortillas, and other, denser baked goods that are not going to have a fluffy texture. Lighter flours, such as white rice flour, tapioca flour, coconut or almond flours, and sweet rice flour, are better for cake batters and cookies.

"Gluten-free baking is always a struggle with texture," she says. "It is very important to realize that you will have stickier doughs, and you will need to use plastic wrap or other tools to work it that normally are not needed in regular baking."

Working gluten-free takes trial and error—and a lot of patience. "Failures are okay, we all have them," says Donna.

This chapter leads off with the recipes Donna has graciously contributed to this book, including several of the recipes made famous at her café, her private gluten-free flour blend, and others she developed expressly for this book, such as a gluten-free pizza crust made out of—are you ready for this?—*potatoes!*

The other recipes come from parents from our Brain Balance community who understand all too well about the trial and error of working with gluten-free flours. Thanks to all of them, you'll see smiles on your child's face instead of tears. Gone are the days of making separate baked goods to please every member of your household. These are treats the whole family can enjoy.

ART CAFÉ'S GLUTEN-FREE BREAD[1]

"If there's one thing I know for sure, it's that people who have any type of gluten intolerance will search high and low for bread," says professional baker and restaurateur Donna Gordon-Teixeria. After many tries at coming up with a super-tasting bread—"many failed attempts that came out like bricks or tasted like sawdust"— Donna hit the jackpot with this recipe, which she so graciously is sharing with all of us. Thank you, Donna!

Makes 1 loaf

1 tablespoon dry active yeast
1½ tablespoons granulated sugar
1¼ cups warm water
1⅓ cups rice flour
⅔ cup sorghum flour or tapioca flour
½ cup potato starch
½ cup cornstarch
⅓ cup vegetable oil
3 eggs or equivalent of Donna's Egg Replacer (page 184)
1 tablespoon xanthan gum
1 teaspoon sea salt or regular salt

1. Preheat the oven to 375°F.

2. Grease a 9 x 5-inch loaf pan.

3. In a small bowl dissolve the yeast and sugar in the warm water. Let stand until the yeast softens and begins to form a creamy foam, 5 to 10 minutes.

4. Combine the yeast mixture, rice flour, sorghum flour, potato starch, cornstarch, vegetable oil, eggs, xanthan gum, and salt in the bowl of an electric mixer. Mix on medium speed until incorporated, about 2 minutes.

---

1 Do not use this recipe if you find that your child is sensitive to yeast.

5. Spoon the dough into the prepared loaf pan. Smooth the top of the dough with the back of a wet spoon. Place in a warm place in the kitchen until it has risen just over the top of the loaf pan, about 1 hour. If your kitchen is not warm or is drafty, cover it lightly with a dish towel.

6. Bake until the loaf is medium golden-brown, about 25 minutes.

THE EASIEST EGG REPLACER AROUND

Eggs and baking practically go together, so when you can't have eggs in your diet it makes baking a real challenge! There are plenty of egg replacers available, but none are quite as handy and easy to use as this one, developed by professional baker Donna Gordon-Teixeira, a volunteer with Generation Rescue who created it to help out kids with food sensitivities. This egg replacer makes life easier for parents because you can mix up the batch dry and store it in the refrigerator or freezer. When you're ready to bake, just scoop out what you need and bring to room temperature. The batch makes enough to replace from 45 to 50 eggs.

DONNA'S EGG REPLACER

To make the mixture, combine:

1½ cups tapioca starch
⅔ cups baking powder
⅓ cups baking soda

When ready to bake, keep in mind:

1 egg = ½ tablespoon replacer powder mixed with
    2 tablespoons of water
1 egg yolk = ½ tablespoon replacer powder mixed with
    1 tablespoon of water

Donna adds that she's had great success making thick egg-white meringue by whipping the egg replacer with less water at high speed. To try it, substitute the eggs called for in your recipe with the amount of egg replacer as instructed above, but start with very little water, adding more as you go along. All told, you will use less water. "It takes practice but it does work!" Donna says.

BASIC ALL-OCCASION CAKE

"Kids shouldn't have to miss out on the fun of a birthday cake or other celebration just because they are eating a gluten-free diet," says Donna Gordon-Teixeira, who developed this recipe for the children of her celebrity clients. It's a basic recipe that can be made into any kind of a cake, from birthday to wedding. She also uses it for cupcakes. "It layers well, and if you add cocoa powder it can become a chocolate cake in a snap," she says. Add the amount of cocoa powder that will suit your family's taste. You can also serve it as a trifle by layering in coco whip and fresh fruit.

Makes one 19 x 13-inch sheet cake, two 9-inch rounds, or about 24 cupcakes

¼ cup coconut flour
2¾ cups Donna's GF All-Purpose Flour (page 188), plus more for the pan
1⅔ cups granulated sugar
1 tablespoon baking powder
½ teaspoon sea salt
¾ cup Earth Balance vegan butter, softened but not melted
½ cup vegetable oil or oil of choice (but not olive oil)
8 egg whites or Donna's Egg Replacer for 4 eggs (page 184)
1¼ cups rice, coconut, or almond milk
2 teaspoons pure vanilla extract

1. Preheat the oven to 350°F.

2. Grease and flour the cake pan(s). Cut parchment paper the size of the pans and place on the bottoms to prevent sticking. For cupcakes, line the tins with paper liners.

3. Put the flours, sugar, baking powder, and salt in an electric mixer and beat on low speed until fluffy. Add the butter and oil and continue to mix for about another minute, until incorporated. Add the egg whites and mix until blended well.

4. Add the milk and vanilla a little at a time while mixing on low speed, then switch to high speed and beat for 2 minutes more. The batter should look thick and fluffy.

5. Pour the mixture into the prepared pan(s) and bake for 20 minutes, or until a toothpick inserted in the center comes out clean. For cupcakes, bake for 15 minutes. Cool completely and top with your frosting of choice.

CHEESY DROP ROLLS[2]

Donna Gordon-Teixeira developed this recipe to fill the ever-increasing demand for children who love cheese. "I found a way to incorporate a great dairy-free and casein-free cheese in the gluten-free drop biscuits I used to make for my bakery. The result was nothing short of amazing," she says. She suggests serving these rolls with pasta or soup. If you are eliminating eggs, substitute Donna's Egg Replacer (page 184) and omit the egg whites.

Makes 1 dozen rolls

½ cup white rice flour
½ cup sorghum flour
¼ cup millet flour

---

2 Do not use this recipe if you find that your child is sensitive to yeast.

¼ cup tapioca flour

¼ cup cornstarch

2 teaspoons xanthan gum

1 package active dry yeast

1 teaspoon sea salt

2 tablespoons flaxseed meal

2 whole eggs, at room temperature

2 egg whites, at room temperature

1 cup warm water

2 tablespoons vegetable or canola oil

2 tablespoons honey

2 tablespoons apple cider vinegar

½ cup Daiya dairy-free shredded cheese

1. Combine the flours, cornstarch, xanthan gum, yeast, salt, and flaxseed meal in a medium bowl with a wire whisk.

2. Combine the eggs, egg whites, water, oil, honey, and vinegar in a large bowl. Using a hand mixer set on low or medium speed, beat until the mixture gets frothy. When fully combined, slowly add the dry-ingredient mixture, scraping down the sides of the bowl. Mix until fully blended, with no lumps.

3. Line a cookie sheet with parchment paper. Using a large spoon covered with oil (because the dough is sticky), drop the dough in spoonfuls on the sheet, about an inch apart.

4. Cut a piece of plastic wrap the size of the cookie sheet and spray with nonstick cooking spray. Lay it over the dough balls.

5. Preheat the oven to 200°F. Turn the oven off as soon as it reaches temperature. Immediately put the dough in the oven and let it rise for 90 minutes. Do not open the oven.

6. Remove the plastic wrap, sprinkle the dough with the cheese, and increase the temperature to 350°F. Bake for 30 minutes, or until the crust is golden-brown.

DO-IT-YOURSELF GLUTEN-FREE FLOUR

Restaurateur and professional baker Donna Gordon-Teixeira has perfected the art of gluten-free baking and has become quite famous among gluten-free celebrities and other followers, especially in Southern California. Anyone who has ever tried using gluten-free flour knows that it can be a challenge to make goodies that measure up to "the real thing" in taste and texture. It also requires practiced skill.

Donna invented and perfected this gluten-free all-purpose flour blend when she operated the Art Café, a well-known bakery and lunchtime hot spot in San Luis Obispo that featured gluten-free pastries and bread. Donna's well-guarded secret recipe is her gracious gift toward helping special-needs children who can't tolerate gluten in their diet.

"This will allow parents and others the freedom to substitute this for the all-purpose flour in the recipes featured in this book and family recipes," she says. "It doesn't give off the unpleasant aftertaste inherent in other gluten-free flours. And it will also save money, as gluten-free flour is quite a bit more expensive than regular flour. Enjoy!"

DONNA'S GF ALL-PURPOSE FLOUR

Makes 9 cups

4 cups brown rice flour
2 cups sweet white sorghum flour or white rice flour[3]
2 cups potato starch

---

3   For a lighter blend, use white rice flour.

½ cup tapioca flour or starch (goes by both names, depending on the brand)
½ cup cornstarch[4]
5 teaspoons xanthan gum

Put all of the ingredients in a bowl and sift well. Store in the freezer in an airtight container. Always bring the flour to room temperature before using it in baking.

POTATO PIZZA CRUST[5]

Talk about a novel stand-in for wheat flour—pizza crust made out of potatoes! "I came up with the idea one night when I couldn't sleep," says Donna Gordon-Teixeira. "It's really been a big hit." A potato ricer is a must.

Makes 4 small or 2 medium pizzas

2 large russet potatoes, boiled in skin until fork-tender
⅓ cup water, boiled to 110°F
2 teaspoons agave syrup or honey
One ¼-ounce package active dry yeast
1 cup white rice flour
½ cup tapioca starch
¾ teaspoon kosher salt
1 large egg white
3 tablespoons olive oil

1. When the potatoes are cool enough to handle, gently peel the skins off and work the potatoes through a potato ricer. You want enough to measure 2 cups.

---

4 For those with a corn sensitivity, substitute ½ cup tapioca flour or starch, or arrowroot.
5 Do not make this recipe if you find that your child is sensitive to yeast.

2. Stir together the hot water, agave, and yeast in a small bowl and let this sit for about 5 minutes. If the water is the correct temperature, a foam will develop. If it does not, discard the liquid and start over with new yeast until you get foam.

3. Fix a stand mixer with a paddle attachment. Add the potatoes, rice flour, tapioca starch, and salt and mix until it forms a fine crumble. Add the egg white and oil.

4. Slowly add in the foamy yeast mixture until it comes together. It will have a tacky consistency. At this point cover the bowl with plastic wrap and place it in a warm area for 1½ hours, or until the dough doubles in size.

5. Remove the dough and form into 4 balls for small pizzas or 2 balls for medium pizzas. Or the dough can be frozen at this stage and thawed out for later use.

TONY'S PIZZA DOUGH[6]

Tony T., a dad at the Brain Balance Achievement Center in Wake Forest, North Carolina, couldn't bear depriving his son of one of his favorite foods when they found out he was sensitive to gluten, so Tony experimented on his own and came up with this gluten-free pizza dough that his family just loves.

Makes one 13-inch pie crust

One ¼-ounce package active dry yeast
1 cup warm water (110°F as measured on a candy thermometer)
2½ cups all-purpose gluten-free flour
½ cup almond flour
2 tablespoons olive oil
1 teaspoon sea salt
2 to 3 tablespoons honey, depending on how sweet you want it
2 teaspoons dried oregano
2 teaspoons dried basil

---

6   Do not make this recipe if you find that your child is sensitive to yeast.

1. Preheat the oven to 350°F.

2. In a small bowl dissolve the yeast in the warm water and let stand until foamy, about 10 minutes.

3. Add the remaining ingredients plus the yeast mixture to a large bowl and knead by hand until the dough is very sticky but not elastic. Cover with plastic wrap and let the dough rise in a warm environment for about 30 minutes.

4. Turn the dough out on a well-floured surface. Flour your hands to work with the dough and prevent it from sticking. If the dough is too sticky, add a bit more gluten-free flour. Be careful not to add too much or it will make a crust that is too dry.

5. Form the dough into a round and, using a rolling pin, press it into a pizza-crust shape. It will make a ¼-inch crust. Place the dough on a pizza stone and top with your favorite sauce and toppings. Bake until golden-brown, about 20 minutes.

APPLE CARROT CAKE

This cake was offered at an open house at the Brain Balance Achievement Center in Bluffton, South Carolina, and it was a huge hit. All the parents wanted the recipe. Director Heather Lowenthal says this recipe was made with Better Batter Gluten-Free Flour Blend, which contains xanthan gum.

Makes 1 cake

2 cups gluten-free flour blend
¾ cup shredded carrots
¾ cup unsweetened applesauce
¾ cup coconut oil, olive oil, or melted butter
¾ cup milk with 1 teaspoon vinegar or lemon juice
1 teaspoon baking powder
1 teaspoon baking soda
1 teaspoon pure vanilla extract
½ teaspoon sea salt

1. Preheat the oven to 350°F.

2. Combine all of the ingredients in a large bowl and thoroughly blend by hand. Transfer to a 9 x 9-inch greased cake pan. Bake for 30 to 45 minutes, or until a toothpick inserted in the center comes out clean. Cool the cake for 20 to 30 minutes before taking it out of the pan.

SO-EASY CHOCOLATE BROWNIES

Brownies are always a crowd pleaser, and this recipe is so quick and easy, even your kids can make them. These brownies were a hit at Donna Gordon-Teixeira's Art Café, and she still makes them at home today. They're equally good with or without frosting. For a super-smart shortcut, Donna suggests putting the first six ingredients in a Ziploc bag, writing the last three ingredients on the outside of the bag, then storing it in your pantry until the time arises to make them. You can also put the dry ingredients in mason jars with the recipe attached and give them out as holiday gifts. For added crunch, fold in ½ to 1 cup broken pecan or walnuts to the mixture.

Makes about 1 dozen brownies

> ½ cup Donna's GF All-Purpose Flour (page 188)
> ⅓ cup baking cocoa
> 1 cup granulated sugar
> ¼ teaspoon sea salt
> ¼ teaspoon baking powder
> ½ cup semisweet chocolate chips or chunks
> 2 eggs or equivalent of Donna's Egg Replacer (page 184)
> ½ cup vegetable or canola oil
> 1 teaspoon pure vanilla extract

1. Preheat the oven to 350°F.

2. Grease an 8 x 8-inch or 9 x 9-inch baking pan and set aside.

3. In a large bowl mix together the flour, cocoa, sugar, salt, and baking powder. Add the chocolate chips, eggs, oil, and vanilla and mix well by

hand with a rubber spatula for 2 to 3 minutes. Scrape into the prepared pan and bake for 12 to 15 minutes, or until a toothpick inserted in the center comes out clean.

DARK CHOCOLATE BROWNIES

Clare B., a Brain Balance mom, shared her recipe for gluten-free brownies with other families at the achievement center in Minnetonka, Minnesota. Everyone wanted the recipe! Here it is.

Makes 16 brownies

5 ounces high-quality 60% to 70% dark chocolate
½ cup coconut oil
1 cup light brown sugar, not packed
½ cup almond meal
¼ cup sorghum flour
½ teaspoon fine sea salt
¼ teaspoon baking soda
2 free-range eggs, beaten
1 tablespoon bourbon vanilla extract
½ cup chopped pecans or walnuts (optional)
Dark chocolate chips, for the top (optional)

1. Preheat the oven to 350°F.

2. Melt the dark chocolate and coconut oil in a saucepan over low heat, stirring gently. (Or melt in a microwave-safe measuring cup and stir together to combine.)

3. In a mixing bowl whisk together the brown sugar, almond meal, sorghum flour, salt, and baking soda. Make a well in the center and add the beaten eggs, vanilla extract, and melted dark-chocolate mixture. Beat on low-medium speed for 2 minutes, until the batter begins to come together. At first it will seem thin, like cake batter, but keep beating until it thickens and becomes smooth and glossy. If you are adding nuts, stir them in by hand.

4. Line an 8 x 8-inch baking pan with parchment paper so that the

paper extends slightly over the sides. Spread the batter in the pan. Sprinkle the top with the chocolate chips and press in lightly, if using. Bake for 30 to 35 minutes, or until the brownies are set. The top will crack like a flourless cake.

5. Cool on a wire rack for 1 hour. Cut into 16 pieces. Remove by lifting the brownies out of the pan by the ends of the parchment paper.

ART CAFÉ BANANA BREAD

Though Donna Gordon-Teixeira no longer operates her Art Café, she still gets called on to make her famous banana bread. "I'm still making multiple loaves and passing them on to friends, clients, and family," she says. "People tell me all the time that they have no idea that it is gluten free." The key to great taste, she says, is to use to very ripe bananas. Wait until they are almost black.

Makes 1 loaf

2 cups Donna's GF All-Purpose Flour (page 188)
1 teaspoon baking soda
1 teaspoon baking powder
½ teaspoon ground cinnamon
¼ teaspoon sea salt
½ cup Earth Balance butter
1 cup granulated sugar
2 eggs or equivalent of Donna's Egg Replacer (page 184)
1 teaspoon pure vanilla extract
1½ cups very ripe mashed bananas (about 4 or 5 bananas)

1. Preheat the oven to 350°F.

2. Lightly grease a 9 x 5-inch loaf pan and set aside.

3. In a large bowl combine the flour, baking soda, baking powder, cinnamon, and salt.

4. In another large bowl cream together the butter and sugar. Stir in the eggs and vanilla. Stir in the bananas, just until blended.

5. Add the flour mixture to the banana mixture and stir just until moistened. Do not overmix. You can also stir in nuts or dried fruits, or any other addition you desire.

6. Pour in the loaf pan and smooth with a rubber spatula. Bake for 50 to 60 minutes, or until a toothpick inserted into the center of the loaf comes out clean. Cool on a wire rack for 10 minutes before removing from the pan.

ART CAFÉ BLUEBERRY MUFFINS

Nothing is more pleasant than the smell of fresh baked muffins in the morning. This quick-and-easy gluten-free muffin recipe was a hit at Donna Gordon-Teixeira's Art Café. The best part is that you can swap out the blueberries for any fruit, dried fruit, or nuts. The secret to fluffy muffins, says Donna, is to not mix them too hard. Overmixing produces dense muffins.

Makes 1 dozen muffins

    1 stick Earth Balance butter
    1 large egg or equivalent of Donna's Egg Replacer (page 184)
    1 teaspoon pure vanilla extract
    1 cup full-fat coconut milk, rice milk, or almond milk
    2 cups Donna's GF All-Purpose Flour (page 188)
    ½ cup plus 2 teaspoons raw sugar
    1 tablespoon baking powder
    ½ teaspoon sea salt
    1 cup fresh or frozen blueberries

1. Preheat the oven to 375°F.

2. Melt the butter in a small pan over medium heat and set aside to cool. Transfer to a small bowl. Add the egg, vanilla, and milk and beat with a wire whisk until well blended. Set aside.

3. In a large mixing bowl combine the flour, ½ cup sugar, baking powder, and salt with a table fork. Add the liquid ingredients and the blueberries to the flour mixture using a rubber spatula. Mix lightly to blend.

4. Line 12 muffin tins with paper liners and spoon equal amounts of batter into the cups. Sprinkle the tops with the remaining 2 teaspoons sugar. Bake for 18 to 20 minutes, or until the tops are brown and a toothpick inserted in the center comes out clean. Cool on a wire rack for about 15 minutes before removing from the pan.

GRAHAM CRACKER COOKIES

Remember Teddy Grahams? Well, these are better. "We passed them around at the center one day and everyone was asking Carrie T., the mom who made them, for the recipe," says Heather Lowenthal, of the achievement center in Bluffton, South Carolina. "What a hit!" You can make chocolate graham cracker cookies by substituting ½ cup of unsweetened cocoa for ½ cup of the gluten-free flour. These cookies have a softer feel than traditional graham crackers.

Makes about 2 dozen, depending on the size of the cookie cutter

> 2½ cups gluten-free flour, such as Donna's GF All-Purpose Flour (page 188)
> ½ cup palm sugar
> ½ teaspoon sea salt
> 1 teaspoon ground cinnamon
> 1 teaspoon baking soda
> ½ cup softened butter
> ¼ cup honey
> ¼ cup water

1. Preheat the oven to 350°F.

2. Put the flour, sugar, salt, cinnamon, and baking soda in the bowl of a food processor and pulse until thoroughly mixed.

3. Add the butter and pulse until completely incorporated. Add the honey and water and mix until a dough forms.

4. Remove from the food processor and roll into a disk ¼-inch thick. Using a cookie cutter, cut into shapes of gingerbread men or whatever

shape you prefer. Place them on a greased cookie sheet. Bake for 15 minutes, or until they are completely cooked. Store them in an airtight container for up to 7 days.

ART CAFÉ GLUTEN-FREE CHOCOLATE-CHIP COOKIES

What kid doesn't like chocolate-chip cookies, and what parent doesn't like making them! It only gets challenging when the cookies have to be gluten free. In this recipe Donna Gordon-Teixeira uses Earth Balance as the butter substitute because it is vegan and dairy free.

Makes about 2 dozen cookies

2 cups rice flour, brown or white
¾ cup sorghum flour
½ cup tapioca starch
2 teaspoons xanthan gum
1 teaspoon baking soda
1 teaspoon sea salt
1 cup Earth Balance spread, softened to room temperature
¾ cup granulated sugar, natural cane or raw
¾ cup light brown sugar, natural or raw
1 teaspoon pure vanilla extract
2 eggs or equivalent of Donna's Egg Replacer (page 184)
1½ cups chocolate chips (or more if you like)

1. Preheat the oven to 350°F.

2. In a medium bowl combine the rice flour, sorghum flour, tapioca starch, xanthan gum, baking soda, and salt. Set aside.

3. In the bowl of an electric mixer set on medium speed, cream together the Earth Balance spread, sugars, and vanilla until light and fluffy, 2 to 3 minutes. Add the eggs until just combined. Do not overmix.

4. Turn the mixer to low speed and add the dry ingredients to the creamed ingredients until they are well combined, about 3 minutes. Re-

duce the speed to low and add the chocolate chips until they are well distributed in the dough.

5. Line a cookie sheet with parchment paper. Drop the cookies by rounded spoonfuls or make round balls. Refrigerate for 5 minutes to prevent spread.

6. Bake for 10 minutes. Remove and allow to cool on the sheet for 5 minutes, as they will continue to bake while cooling.

DONNA'S GLUTEN-FREE PIE CRUST AND PIE FILLINGS

"The secret to a perfect gluten-free pie crust is to roll it out between two pieces of plastic wrap," says Donna Gordon-Teixeira. "This way it doesn't stick and you don't have to add extra flour, which will dry out the crust." She uses Earth Balance butter and Spectrum shortening in this recipe because they are both gluten- and casein-free. The crust freezes well and will keep for six months. For the total pie experience, top these pie fillings with So Delicious CocoWhip nondairy whip topping.

Makes 1 crust

PIE CRUST
1½ cups Donna's GF All-Purpose Flour (page 188)
2 tablespoons granulated sugar
½ teaspoon sea salt
4 tablespoons cold Earth Balance spread
3 tablespoons nonhydrogenated shortening, such as Spectrum
4 tablespoons ice-cold water
1 teaspoon apple cider vinegar

1. In a large bowl sift together the flour, sugar, and salt. Add the Earth Balance spread and shortening, using a pastry cutter or two forks. Combine until the ingredients resemble coarse crumbs and the butter pieces are less than pea-size.

2. Add the water and cider vinegar and continue to blend until it reaches a doughy consistency. Add another tablespoon of water, if necessary. Pat the dough into a round disc and place in plastic wrap in the refrigerator for at least 1 hour.

3. Cut two pieces of plastic wrap about 15 inches long. Lay one piece of the wrap on a flat rolling surface. Place the cold disc of dough in the center. Top with the second piece of plastic wrap. Roll out a 13-inch round with a rolling pin. Carefully remove the plastic wrap from the top and flip the crust into a greased pie tin. Remove the last piece of plastic wrap, pressing together any cracks that form. Crimp the edges. The crust is now ready for its filling.

PUMPKIN FILLING

    2 cups unsweetened pumpkin puree

    1 cup full-fat coconut milk, such as So Delicious Culinary Coconut Milk, stirred

    ½ cup cane sugar or honey for a different taste

    2 tablespoons pure maple syrup (omit this if you use honey)

    1 teaspoon pure vanilla extract

    ¼ cup cornstarch (use tapioca starch for corn sensitivity or for preference)

    1 teaspoon ground cinnamon

    ½ teaspoon ground ginger

    ¼ teaspoon ground nutmeg

1. Preheat the oven to 350°F.

2. Put all of the ingredients in a large bowl and combine well. Pour into Donna's GF Pie Crust and bake for 50 to 55 minutes.

APPLE FILLING[7]

> 6 cups peeled and thinly sliced Granny Smith apples
>
> ¾ cup granulated sugar
>
> 1 tablespoon fresh lemon juice
>
> 1 teaspoon ground cinnamon
>
> ¼ teaspoon ground nutmeg

1. Preheat the oven to 425°F.

2. Put the apples in a large mixing bowl. Add the remaining ingredients and mix thoroughly. Pour into Donna's GF Pie Crust. Top with a second pie crust and crimp the edges together. Cut a few slits into the top crust. Bake for 40 minutes.

---

7 Do not use this filling if you find that your child is sensitive to apples.

Chapter 11
Snacks That Don't Attack

The eternal fight over junk food *can* come to a halt. And guess what: Sugar isn't as bad as some parents are led to believe. As I explained in Chapter 3, you needn't worry about giving your child a *reasonable amount* of sugar—that means an occasional treat—unless your child has a problem with metabolizing sugar and other simple carbohydrates, which is something your child's doctor can assess. However, most of the snacks you find in stores qualify as junk food, which is why Brain Balance nutritionists and parents go the extra mile to come up with ideas for healthier snacks they can make for their kids in their own kitchens. Here are some of their ideas.

HEALTHIER GRANOLA BARS

Granola sounds healthy, but not if you have food sensitivities. Stacey Gadbois of Virginia Beach, Virginia, has remedied that with this version, which avoids gluten, yeast, soy, corn, dairy, and refined sugar. "The options for making these are endless," she says, "and kids love to snack on them." You can add up to a ½ cup of all or any of these ingredients without changing the consistency: unsweetened coconut flakes, slivered almonds, chopped nuts, or whole seeds. Make sure the peanut butter is mixed well. If it is too oily, she says, the bars will not set.

Makes 8 bars

¾ cup natural peanut butter
1 ripe banana, mashed
½ cup clarified butter or coconut oil
1 teaspoon pure vanilla extract

    ¼ cup coconut sugar

    ¼ cup xylitol

    ½ teaspoon sea salt

    2½ cups gluten-free rolled oats

    ½ cup pumpkin seeds

    1 cup unsulfured raisins

    ½ cup flaxseeds

    ½ cup dark (dairy-free) chocolate chips

1. Preheat the oven to 350°F.

2. Put the peanut butter, mashed banana, butter, vanilla, coconut sugar, and xylitol in a large bowl and beat with an electric mixer on low speed until smooth and well combined. Add the remaining ingredients and stir with a spoon.

3. Grease an 8 x 8-inch baking pan with nonstick spray. Add the granola mixture. Bake for 30 minutes. Cool, cover, and refrigerate for at least 2 hours before cutting. Cut into 2-inch squares. Store refrigerated. The longer they are refrigerated, the firmer they will be.

CHERRY-COCONUT POWER BARS

These protein bars can often be found at North Carolina's Brain Balance Achievement Center, which serves Midlothian, Virginia, and Cary and Chapel Hill, North Carolina, where they are given out as treats to the kids and their families to sample. The parents like to keep them handy on outings when children get hungry. They also pack well in school lunch boxes. For a change of flavor, you can substitute raisins for the cherries.

Makes about 30 bars

    3½ cups gluten-free oats

    ¾ cup dried cherries

    ⅔ cup sunflower seeds

    ½ cup toasted sesame seeds

    1 cup quinoa flakes

3 tablespoons ground flaxseeds
1 cup unsweetened shredded coconut (optional)
1 cup chocolate chips (optional)
1 tablespoon ground cinnamon
1 teaspoon sea salt
2 cups almond butter or sunflower butter
1¾ cups pure maple syrup
½ cup coconut oil

1. Preheat the oven to 350°F.

2. In a large bowl combine the oats, cherries, sunflower seeds, quinoa, flaxseeds, coconut, chocolate chips, cinnamon, and salt. Set aside.

3. Mix the almond butter, maple syrup, and coconut oil in a small saucepan over low heat and cook until bubbly. Pour over the dry ingredients and mix well.

4. Press the mixture into a greased 9 x 13-inch baking sheet and bake for 15 to 20 minutes, or until slightly firm to the touch. Cool completely before cutting into 2-inch squares. Wrap individually in plastic wrap and store in the refrigerator. You can pull out one when needed. These also freeze very well.

SULFITE ALERT

For those sensitive to sulfite: Packaged grated coconut is sometimes preserved using sulfites, so check the label carefully before buying. Better yet, grate your own, recommends Christie Korth, Brain Balance corporate nutrition director.

ALMOND-PEANUT BUTTER PROTEIN BALLS

This snack helps fill in the nutritional gaps common to many children who visit Brain Balance. Each treat contains 7 grams of protein and about 16 milligrams of calcium—and kids love them. The recipe is courtesy of the Brain Balance Achievement Center in Tulsa, Oklahoma. Be sure to use only organic natural peanut butter.

Makes about 1 dozen balls

> 1 cup almond flour
> 1 scoop rice or pea protein, such as Now Foods unflavored or NutriBiotic plain rice protein
> ¼ cup chia seeds
> ½ cup almond butter
> 2 tablespoons natural peanut butter
> 2 tablespoons agave nectar
> 2 tablespoons pure maple sugar
> ¼ cup sunflower seeds or unsweetened coconut flakes

1. Combine all of the ingredients except the sunflower seeds or coconut flakes in the bowl of a food processor and pulse until mixed, about 1 minute.

2. Scoop about a tablespoon into the palms of your hands and roll into a ball. Roll in the seeds or coconut to cover.

3. Transfer to a plastic container in a single layer. Repeat with each ball. Refrigerate, covered, for at least 1 hour before serving. Store in the refrigerator for up to 2 weeks.

PEANUT BUTTER CHOCOLATE-CHIP COOKIE BALLS

Casey Rhoads shares this recipe with the families who come to the Brain Balance Achievement Center in Glassboro, New Jersey, where she is the program director. Kids love them for their peanuty-chocolaty taste. You'd never guess they're made with chickpeas instead of flour! They are best served warm and gooey, so pop them into a hot oven or microwave for a minute or two before serving. Make sure to use natural peanut butter or the recipe won't work.

Makes about 1 dozen

1¼ cups canned chickpeas, drained
2 teaspoons pure vanilla extract
½ cup plus 2 tablespoons natural peanut butter
¼ cup honey
1 teaspoon baking powder
Pinch salt
½ cup chocolate chips

1. Preheat the oven to 350°F.

2. Rinse and pat dry the chickpeas. Add the chickpeas and the rest of the ingredients, except the chocolate chips, to the bowl of a food processor and blend until smooth. Fold in the chocolate chips. The consistency should be thick and sticky.

3. Line a cookie sheet with parchment paper. Moisten your hands, roll the dough into 1-inch balls, and place them on the cookie sheet. Bake for 10 minutes. They will come out soft rather than hard like regular cookies. Store in an airtight container at room temperature or in the refrigerator. They will keep for about a week.

PEANUT BUTTER FUDGE

"I grew up on homemade fudge, so perfecting this recipe to avoid food-sensitivity issues was near bliss," says Stacey Gadbois.

Makes 8 servings

2 cans full-fat coconut milk
½ cup xylitol
1 teaspoon pure vanilla extract
3 cups dairy-free semisweet chocolate chips
⅛ teaspoon sea salt
1½ cups natural peanut butter

1. Line an 8-inch square baking pan crisscrossed with two pieces of 10-inch-square parchment paper, so you have a 2-inch overhang on both sides. The overhanging edges will serve as handles to lift the fudge from the pan.

2. Put the coconut milk and xylitol in a medium saucepan over medium-high heat and bring to a boil. Continue boiling, stirring constantly, until the mixture is reduced by half, about 5 to 10 minutes.

3. Remove the pan from the heat and add the vanilla, chocolate chips, and salt. Stir until smooth. Add the peanut butter and mix well. Pour the fudge into the pan and spread evenly. Refrigerate for at least 4 hours. Cut into 2-inch-square pieces. Keep refrigerated.

CHOCOLATE-CHIP PEANUT BUTTER CRISPS[1]

When the sweet tooth calls, these crisps are the answer. Parents at the Brain Balance Achievement Center in Bluffton, South Carolina, rave over this healthy alternative to candy.

Makes 12 to 15 treats

One 10-ounce box brown rice cereal
1¾ cups brown rice syrup
Pinch salt
¾ cup natural peanut butter
½ cup chocolate chips or dairy-free chocolate chips

1. Pour the rice cereal into a mixing bowl.

2. Heat the brown rice syrup with the salt in a medium saucepan over medium heat until it becomes a loose liquid. When the syrup is pourable, stir in the peanut butter until well blended.

3. Pour the liquid mixture over the rice cereal and blend well. Set aside to cool.

4. When cool, stir in the chocolate chips. Pour into an 8 x 8-inch or 9 x 13-inch baking pan. Press the mixture into the pan. Place in the refrigerator for 1 hour to cool, then cut into squares. Store in an airtight container. The crisps will keep for 3 to 5 days but will disappear long before that!

---

1 If your child is sensitive to chocolate, you can substitute carob.

CHOCOLATE-PEANUT BUTTER SWIRL CUPS

A healthier, richer alternative to a peanut butter cup, courtesy of Stacey Gadbois. Always serve them cold (and with a napkin), as they melt quickly. If a peanut allergy is on your list, you can substitute almond or cashew butter.

Makes 1 dozen cups

1 cup natural peanut butter
½ tablespoon coconut oil
1 tablespoon xylitol
½ cup unsweetened shredded coconut
Pinch salt
1 cup dairy-free chocolate chips, melted

1. Put the peanut butter, coconut oil, xylitol, coconut, and salt in a blender and blend until smooth.

2. Spray a mini-muffin pan with nonstick spray. Drop a spoonful of peanut butter mixture into each tin. Drop half a spoonful of the melted chocolate on top of the peanut butter mixture and swirl with a toothpick. Place in the freezer for 1 hour. Remove the candies with a sharp knife. Refrigerate or freeze to keep.

OATMEAL CHOCOLATE-CHIP COOKIES[2]

Melissa D., a Brain Balance mom at the Edwardsville, IL, Brain Balance Center, came up with this recipe for healthy cookies containing lots of yummy ingredients kids will love—bananas, nuts, applesauce, and, of course, chocolate chips. And it's so easy.

Makes 25 to 30 cookies

3 very ripe medium bananas, mashed
⅓ cup unsweetened applesauce
2 cups gluten-free rolled oats

---

2   Do not use this recipe if you find that your child is sensitive to apples.

¼ cup raisins or chopped nuts (optional)
¼ cup unsweetened vanilla almond milk
1 cup dark or semisweet chocolate chips
1 teaspoon pure vanilla extract
1 teaspoon ground cinnamon
¼ cup brown sugar (optional)

1. Preheat the oven to 350°F.

2. Put all of the ingredients in a large mixing bowl and combine well with a fork.

3. Line a nonstick cookie sheet with parchment paper. Using a tablespoon, scoop the mixture onto the sheet, keeping the cookies about 2 inches apart. Slightly flatten out each cookie mixture with the back of a fork. Bake for 15 to 20 minutes. Allow the cookies to cool for a few minutes before attempting to remove them from the sheet.

POWER POPSICLES

These frozen pops are a big hit at the Brain Balance Achievement Center in Wake Forest, North Carolina. They're a quick, easy way to sneak in protein, which plays an important role in brain development and function. And they taste so good your kids won't even realize you're giving them a healthy treat. You can substitute almond or rice milk for the coconut milk, if needed.

Makes 5 to 6 popsicles

One 13.5-ounce can full-fat coconut milk
2 scoops protein powder

Shake the can well. Put the coconut milk in a blender with the protein powder and blend for 20 to 30 seconds. Pour into popsicle molds and freeze.

COCONUT NUT BALLS

Give your kids a protein kick with these special treats, which make an excellent snack or dessert. Make sure to refrigerate them for at least 30 minutes before serving, or they will be too sticky, says Stacey Gadbois.

Makes 8 servings

½ cup brown rice syrup
½ cup natural or raw almonds
¼ cup solid clarified butter, ghee, or coconut oil
1 teaspoon ground cinnamon
½ cup chopped pecans
¾ cup plus ½ cup unsweetened coconut flakes

1. Preheat the oven to 350°F.

2. Pulse the syrup, almonds, clarified butter, and cinnamon in a food processor until the almonds are well chopped. Spray an 8 x 8-inch baking dish with nonstick spray. Spread the mixture into the pan. Sprinkle with the chopped pecans and ¾ cup of the coconut flakes. Bake for 15 minutes. Set aside to cool. Once cooled, refrigerate for at least 4 hours.

3. Remove from the refrigerator and form the mixture into balls about 2 inches round. Roll the balls in the remaining unsweetened coconut. Serve immediately or keep refrigerated. The longer the balls are in the refrigerator, the firmer they will be.

PUMPKIN-COCONUT RICE PUDDING

This pudding features lots of vitamin A and fiber and the wonderful aromas of the warming spices. "This makes the house smell delicious," says Stacey Gadbois, who developed this recipe.

Makes 8 servings

2 cups filtered water
1 cup arborio rice
3 cups full-fat coconut milk
1 cup unsweetened pumpkin puree

    1 teaspoon pure vanilla extract

    ½ cup xylitol

    1 teaspoon ground cinnamon, plus extra for serving

    ¼ teaspoon ground ginger

    ¼ teaspoon ground nutmeg

    ¼ teaspoon sea salt

1. Preheat the oven to 375°F.

2. Bring the water to a boil in a medium saucepan. Stir in the rice and cover. Reduce the heat to low and cook for about 20 minutes. The rice should be fluffy but not watery. Set aside, uncovered.

3. In a large bowl mix together the coconut milk, pumpkin, vanilla, xylitol, cinnamon, ginger, nutmeg, and salt with a wire whisk. Add the hot rice to this mixture and stir well to combine. Transfer the mixture to a deep baking dish. Cover with foil and bake for 50 minutes. If the mixture is still runny, remove the foil and bake for an additional 10 minutes. Remove from the oven and stir to combine. The mixture will thicken as it cools. Sprinkle with cinnamon to serve. Refrigerate once cooled.

BAKED KALE CHIPS

Kale is known as the queen of greens for its super-rich antioxidant and anti-inflammatory properties, and kale chips are all the rage as a healthy alternative to potato chips. "My daughter is a very picky eater and is sensitive to a lot of foods. She just loves this snack," says Stacey Gadbois. "I like the nutritional value it delivers."

Makes 1 large bowlful

    1 bunch kale

    Olive oil spray, such as Misto

    ½ teaspoon sea salt

1. Preheat the oven to 350° F.

2. Rinse the kale and dry it well in a salad spinner. With a knife, remove the leaves from the stems. Discard the stems. Place the leaves on a baking sheet lined with parchment paper. Spray with the olive oil. Sprinkle

with the sea salt and bake until crisp, about 12 minutes. Cool. Store in an airtight container for up to a week.

CHEESY KALE CHIPS[3]

Here's another healthy chip idea with a cheesy twist. These are a family favorite at the Swarthout household in Fresno, California, and a real treat for the staff and children when mom Janeil brings them to the Brain Balance Achievement Center, where she is the executive director. Everyone loves the cheesy taste, even though there is no cheese in them!

Makes 8 to 10 servings

> 2 cups raw cashews
> 3 cups water
> 3 tablespoons raw apple cider vinegar
> Juice of 2 lemons
> 3 red bell peppers, seeded and quartered
> ½ cup nutritional yeast
> 2 cloves garlic, crushed
> 1 large bunch kale

1. Put the cashews in a large bowl. Cover with the water. Stir in 1 tablespoon of the apple cider vinegar and soak for 6 to 8 hours or overnight. Drain and rinse.

2. Put the cashews, lemon juice, and remaining apple cider vinegar in a food processor or a heavy-duty mixer on high speed and process until creamy, about 1 minute. Add the bell peppers, yeast, and garlic and blend again. The mixture should have the consistency of a creamy salad dressing.

3. Wash and dry the kale and remove the stems. Thoroughly coat each kale leaf in the dressing. Add salt to taste. If using a dehydrator, spread the leaves on the dehydrator sheets in a single layer and dehydrate according to the manufacturer's directions for 6 to 8 hours, until crispy. (Times will vary based on the thickness of the coating.) To dry in the

---

3   Skip this recipe if you discover that your child is sensitive to citrus.

oven, spread the leaves on cookie sheets and bake in a 170°F oven for 3 hours, until crispy. Store in a sealable plastic container.

NUTRIENT-PACKED SMOOTHIES

I love smoothies because they are a delicious way to pack a lot of nutrition into a meal or snack. These super-nutritious smoothies were developed by Jordan S. Rubin, Ph.D., author of the *New York Times* bestseller *The Maker's Diet* and most recently *The Maker's Diet Revolution,* and founder of Beyond Organic, a farm-to-consumer company that develops nutrient-dense dairy and other health products.

Rubin believes we have lost our connection to the land and that we are too reliant on chemically laden tap water and food processed to the point that it is unrecognizable. His vision is to reconnect us to the ultimate source of health—food and water from the land, preserved by nature. He designs his products to minimize toxins and maximize nutrition. His recipes, likewise, are designed to do the same. Amasai cultured dairy yogurt can be found at beyondorganic.com. These smoothies work best when made in a high-speed blender. If you don't have one, however, you can use a regular blender for all of the following smoothies, except for those that specifically call for a high-speed blender.

AVOCADO SMOOTHIE

Makes 2 servings

2 very ripe medium bananas
½ avocado
8 ounces plain Amasai cultured dairy yogurt, sheep's milk yogurt, goat's milk yogurt, or coconut milk
2 tablespoons ground chia seeds
1 teaspoon pure vanilla extract
2 cups tightly packed kale or spinach
1 cup cubed or crushed ice

Put all of the ingredients in a blender and blend on high speed until rich and creamy.

BANANA CREAM SMOOTHIE

Makes 2 servings

> 10 ounces plain Amasai cultured dairy yogurt, sheep's milk yogurt, goat's milk yogurt, or coconut milk
> 1 to 2 raw, pastured eggs (optional)
> 1 to 2 tablespoons raw honey
> 1 cup fresh or frozen mashed banana
> ½ teaspoon pure vanilla extract
> 3 tablespoons ground chia seeds

Combine all of the ingredients in a blender and blend until smooth.

SWISS ALMOND-CHOCOLATE SMOOTHIE

Makes 2 servings

> 10 ounces plain Amasai cultured dairy yogurt, goat's milk yogurt, sheep's milk yogurt, or coconut milk
> 1 to 2 raw pastured eggs (optional)
> 1 tablespoon extra-virgin coconut oil
> 1 to 2 tablespoons raw honey
> 2 tablespoons unsweetened cocoa or cacao powder
> 2 tablespoons almond butter
> 1 to 2 fresh or frozen bananas
> ½ teaspoon pure vanilla extract
> 3 tablespoons ground chia seeds

Combine all of the ingredients in a blender and blend until smooth.

TROPICAL SMOOTHIE

Makes 2 servings

> 10 ounces plain Amasai cultured dairy yogurt, sheep's milk yogurt, goat's milk yogurt, or coconut milk
> 2 eggs (optional)
> 1 tablespoon extra-virgin coconut oil

1 to 2 tablespoons raw honey

½ cup fresh or frozen pineapple

½ cup fresh or frozen mango

½ cup fresh or frozen mashed banana

½ teaspoon pure vanilla extract

3 tablespoons chia seeds or flaxseeds (optional)

Combine all of the ingredients in a blender and blend until smooth.

PAPAYA SMOOTHIE

Makes 2 servings

1 small papaya, seeded

1 ripe banana

8 ounces plain Amasai cultured dairy yogurt, sheep's milk yogurt, goat's milk yogurt, or coconut milk

1 cup cubed or crushed ice

Place all of the ingredients in a blender and blend until creamy.

PEACHES-AND-CREAM SMOOTHIE

Makes 2 servings

10 ounces plain Amasai cultured dairy yogurt, sheep's milk yogurt, goat's milk yogurt, or coconut milk

1 to 2 raw, pastured eggs (optional)

1 to 2 tablespoons raw honey

½ to 1 cup fresh or frozen peaches

1 fresh or frozen banana

½ teaspoon pure vanilla extract

Combine all of the ingredients in a high-speed blender and blend until creamy.

TOTAL OMEGA SMOOTHIE

Makes 2 servings

8 ounces plain Amasai cultured dairy yogurt, sheep's milk yogurt, goat's milk yogurt, or coconut milk
2 raw, pastured eggs (optional)
1 medium ripe banana
½ medium avocado
1 tablespoon raw honey
1 tablespoon extra-virgin coconut oil
Dash pure vanilla extract
1 tablespoon EA Live chocolate almonds (optional)
3 tablespoons chia and/or flaxseeds

Combine all of the ingredients in a high-speed blender and blend until smooth.

PIÑA COLADA SMOOTHIE

Makes 2 servings

10 ounces plain Amasai cultured dairy yogurt, sheep's milk yogurt, goat's milk yogurt, or coconut milk
2 raw, pastured eggs (optional)
1 tablespoon extra-virgin coconut oil
1 to 2 tablespoons raw honey
1 cup fresh or frozen pineapple
½ fresh or frozen banana
½ teaspoon pure vanilla extract
3 tablespoons chia and/or flaxseeds (optional)

Combine all of the ingredients in a high-speed blender and blend until smooth.

ACKNOWLEDGMENTS

I would like to thank my many friends and colleagues who helped in the writing of this book, especially Dr. Datis Kharrazian, Christie Korth, Donna Gordon-Teixeira, Jennifer Fugo, and Zac and Shelly Brown. It would not have been possible without the help of the Brain Balance community that so eagerly offered to share their recipes and experiences. Many thanks to you all. I want to thank my professional colleagues, Jordon Rubin and David Gentile, for their contributions. Their interest in promoting clean and organic eating and living is commendable. I would also like to thank my literary agent, Carol Mann, and her wonderful staff, and Marian Lizzi and her staff at Perigee Books/Penguin Random House. It has been a privilege to work with such a wonderful team on all my books. Of course, I would like to thank my editor and friend Debora Yost. I could not have done any of my books without your help and guidance. I look forward to our next adventure together.

RESOURCES

I have been working with children with special needs for more than twenty-five years and have seen the extraordinary changes the Brain Balance Program has made on thousands of kids, many of whom have parents who thought they had run out of options. The self-help program I featured in my first book, *Disconnected Kids*, has helped tens of thousands of parents see remarkable changes in their children on their own. *The Disconnected Kids Nutrition Plan* will help parents and kids take a big step forward, toward even more positive change.

There is still much more to learn about the nutritional needs of special-needs children, and to many parents, the food challenges they face can seem unending. Many of the nutritional techniques that we use at Brain Balance, which are featured in this book, were developed by Brain Balance's corporate nutrition director Christie Korth. Christie also is in private practice as a holistic nutrition counselor. You can find her at happyandhealthywellness.com.

For more information about Brain Balance and the advances we are making, go to our website, www.brainbalancecenters.com. We continually update the site with new developments in our program, the latest in research, and inspiring stories from parents. In addition, we feature self-help tips for parents from time to time, especially advice on conquering food battles.

To find out more about your child's developmental needs, I have launched an interactive site called The Melillo 7-Day Challenge, which you can find at learn.drrobertmelillo.com/assessment/. You can follow the step-by-step process, complete with audio and graphics, online or it can be accessed through your smartphone.

Since the first Brain Balance Achievement Center opened in 2006, we have grown to nearly one hundred locations across the United States, and more centers are being planned. To find a center close to you, visit our website, brainbalancecenters.com. You can reach me directly through this site as well, or you can contact me through my website, drrobertmelillo .com. I'd love to hear from you. You can also keep up with the latest news and findings by following Brain Balance on Facebook. You can also follow me on Facebook and Twitter (@drrobmelillo).

To find out more about functional neurology or to find a functional neurology specialist, visit the International Association of Functional Neurology and Rehabilitation at its website IAFNR.org and Dr. Datis Kharrazian's website for The Institute of Functional Medicine at functionalmedicine .org.

Space did not permit me to go into great detail on everything you need to know to establish a gluten-free household, which can appear daunting at first. I know, as I've done it myself. For more information on how to live gluten free and for gluten-free recipes and cooking tips, you can go to glutenfreeschool.com, which is owned and operated by Jennifer Fugo, whose advice and recipes are featured in this book. Her book, *The Savvy Gluten-Free Shopper,* can be found online.

To contact professional gluten-free pastry chef Donna Gordon-Teixeira with private chef and recipe inquiries, write to her at finallygfree@gmail .com. You can also follow her on Twitter at (@finallygfree). For more information about dairy-free products, go to the website sodeliciousdairyfree.com. To learn more about the revolutionary work in organic living being conducted by Jordon S. Rubin and colleagues at Beyond Organic and for more of his recipes, visit his website beyondorganic.com. Also check out his new venture at getrealnutrition.com, which is dedicated to restoring real food nutrition to the body and vitality to the planet.

To find out more about brain and body wellness through nutrition, visit Dr. David Gentile's website for his clinic Oasis Integrative Medicine at oasismedicine.com.

For more information on how to expand your child's food choices through food chaining, reference the book *Food Chaining* by Cheri Fraker, Mark Fishbein MD, Sibyl Cox, and Laura Walbert.

If you have a child with vision problems who needs to wear glasses, check out the fun frames called Funoogles, which are available at funoogles .com.

Last but certainly not least, to find out more about Zac Brown's Camp Southern Ground, due to open around the same time this book hits the stores, visit campsouthernground.com. This state-of-the-art camp will be free of charge to all special-needs children. Donations will allow for its continued success. I plan to make my proceeds from this book part of that endeavor.

SELECTED REFERENCES

Adams J.B., George F., Audhya T. 2006. Abnormally high plasma levels of vitamin B6 in children with autism not taking supplements compared to controls not taking supplements. *Journal of Alternative and Complementary Medicine.* 12(1):59–63.

Batista-García-Ramó K., Rodríguez-Rojas R., Carballo-Barreda M., Machado C., Melillo R., Leisman G. 2011. Tractography assessment in autism spectrum disorders. Paper presented at the International Symposium of Disorders of Consciousness, Havana, Cuba, December 6–8.

Birch L.L., Fisher J.O., Davison K.K. 2003. Learning to overeat: maternal use of restrictive feeding practices promotes girls' eating in the absence of hunger. *American Journal of Clinical Nutrition.* Sug.;78(2):215–20.

Birch L.L. et al. 1982. Effects of instrumental consumption on children's food preference. *Appetite.* June; 3(2):125–34.

Black M.M. 1998. Zinc deficiency and child development. *American Journal of Clinical Nutrition.* Aug.; 68(2 Suppl): 464S–69S.

Bourre J.M. 2006. Effects of nutrients (in food) on the structure and function of the nervous system: update on dietary requirements for brain. Part 1: micronutrients. *Journal of Nutritional Health and Aging.* Sept.-Oct.;10(5):377–85.

Burgess J.R. et al. 2000. Long-chain polyunsaturated fatty acids in children with attention-deficit hyperactivity disorder. *American Journal of Clinical Nutrition.* Jan.;71(1 Suppl):327S–30S.

Calero C.I. et al. 2001. Allosteric modulation of retinal GABA receptors by ascorbic acid. *Journal of Neuroscience.* June 29;31(26):9672–82.

Cannell J.J., Grant W.B. 2013. What is the role of vitamin D in autism? *Dermato-endocrinology*. Jan. 1;5(1):199–204.

Cavadini C., Siega-Riz A.M., Popkin B.M. 2000. US adolescent food intake trends from 1965 to 1996. *Western Journal of Medicine*. Dec.;173(6):378–83.

Cosar A., Ipcioglu O.M. 2013. Re. Low folate and vitamin B12 nourishment is common in Omani children with newly diagnosed autism. *Nutrition*. Sept.;29(9):1170.

Dolske M.C. et al. 1993. A preliminary trial of ascorbic acid as supplemental therapy for autism. *Progress in Neuro-Psychopharmacology & Biological Psychiatry*. Sept.;17(5):765–74.

Dura-Trave T., Gallinas-Victoriano F. 2014. Caloric and nutrient intake in children with attention deficit hyperactivity disorder treated with extended-release methylphenidate: analysis of a cross-sectional nutrition survey. *JRSM Open*. Feb. 3;5(2):2042533313517690.

Dura-Trave T., Bayona D.V., Petri Y., Albes A. 2014. Dietary patterns in patients with attention deficit hyperactive disorder. *Anales de Pediatría (Barcelona)*. April;80(4):206–13.

Elgar F.J., Craig W., Trites S.J. 2013. Family dinners, communication, and mental health in Canadian adolescents. *Journal of Adolescent Health*. April;52(10):433–38.

Estevez M., Machado C., Leisman G., Melillo R., Machado A., Hernandez-Cruz A., Arias A., Rodriguez-Rojas R., Carballo M. EEGConn. 2013. A software tool for offline qEEG analysis, including spectral univariate and bivariate processes and linear and non-linear indices of brian connectivity in autistic spectrum disorder. *Chronic Disease and Disability in Childhood*. Haupaugue, NY: Nova Scientific, p. 65.

Frensham L.J., Bryan J., Parletta N. 2012. Influences of micronutrient and omega-3 fatty acid supplementation on cognition, learning, and behavior: methodological considerations and implications for children and adolescents in developed societies. *Nutrition Review*. Oct.;70(10):594–610.

Frye R.E., Rossignol D.E. 2014. Treatments for biomedical abnormalities associated with autism spectrum disorder. *Frontiers in Pediatrics*. June 27;2:66.

Galloway A.T. et al. 2005. Parental pressure, dietary patterns, and weight status among girls who are "picky eaters." *Journal of the American Dietetic Association.* April;105(4):541–48.

Garbutt J.M. et al. 2012. What are parents worried about? Health problems and health concerns for children. *Clinical Pediatrics.* Sept.;51(9):840–47.

Grabrucker A.M. 2013. Environmental factors in autism. *Frontiers in Psychiatry.* Jan. 18;3:118.

Grabrucker S. et al. 2014. Zinc deficiency dysregulates the synaptic ProSAP/Shank scaffold and might contribute to autism spectrum disorders. *Brain.* Jan.;137(Pt 1):137–52.

Ghanizadeh A. 2013. Increased glutamate and homocysteine and decreased glutamine levels in autism: a review and strategies for future studies of amino acids in autism. *Disease Markers.* Sept. 12;epub.

Gumpricht E., Rockway S. 2014. Can ω-3 fatty acids and tocotrienol-rich vitamin E reduce symptoms of neurodevelopmental disorders? *Nutrition.* July–Aug.;30(7–8):733–38.

Gvozdjakova A. et al. 2014. Ubiquinol improves symptoms in children with autism. *Oxidative Medicine and Cellular Longevity.* Feb. 23 Epub.

Harrison F.E., May J.M. 2009. Vitamin C function in the brain: vital role of the ascorbate transporter (SVCT2). *Free Radical Biology & Medicine.* Mar. 15;46(6):719–30.

Heilskov R.M. et al. 2014. Diet in the treatment of ADHD in children—A systematic review of the literature. *Nordic Journal of Psychiatry.* June 16:1-18. Epub.

Hyman S.L. et al. 2012. Nutrient intake from food in children with autism. *Pediatrics.*Nov.;130 Suppl 2:S145–53.

The Importance of Family Dinners. 2011. The National Center on Addiction and Substance Abuse at Columbia University.

Jacka F.N. et al. 2011. A prospective study of diet quality and mental health in adolescents. *PloS One.* 6(9):e24805. doi: 10.1371.

Joshi K. et al. 2006. Supplementation with flax oil and vitamin C improves the outcome of Attention Deficit Hyperactivity Disorder (ADHD). *Prostaglandins, Leukotrienes, and Essential Fatty Acids.* Jan.;74(1):17–21.

Kaluzna-Czaplinkska J. et al. 2013. A focus on homocysteine in autism. *Acta biochimica Polonica.* 60(2):137–42.

Kidd P.M. 2002. Autism, an extreme challenge to integrative medicine. Part 2: medical management. *Alternative Medicine Review.* Dec.;7(6):472–99.

Kocovska E. et al. 2014. Vitamin D in the general population of young adults with autism in the Faroe Islands. *Journal of Autism and Developmental Disorders.* June 14. [Epub ahead of print].

Konikowskia K., Regulska-Ilow B., Rozanska D. 2012. The influence of components of diet on the symptoms of ADHD in children. *Roczniki Panstwowego Zakladu Higieny.* 63(2):127–34.

Larsen J.K. et al. 2015. How parental dietary behavior and food parenting practices affect children's dietary behavior. Interacting sources of influence? *Appetite.* June 1;89:246–57.

Leisman G., Braun-Benjamin O., Melillo R. 2014. Cognitive-motor interactions of the basal ganglia in development. *Frontiers in Systems Neuroscience.* 8:16. doi: 10.3389/fnsys.2014.00016. [Cross-referenced in *Frontiers in Computational Neuroscience*].

Leisman G., Melillo R. et al. 2013. Functional disconnectivities in individuals with autistic spectrum disorders. *International Journal of Child Health and Human Development.* 6(4): 486.

Leisman G., Melillo R., Machado C. et al. 2012. Functional disconnectivities in autistic spectrum individuals. Paper presented at the International Conference of Child Health and Human Development, Jerusalem, Israel. December.

Leisman G., Melillo R. 2011. Functional disconnectivities in autistic spectrum disorder as a potent model for explaining disorders of consciousness and cognition in the brain and nervous system. *Functional Neurology, Rehabilitation and Ergonomics.* 1(1);101–45.

Leisman G., Melillo R. et al. 2010. The effect of hemisphere specific remediation strategies on the academic performance outcome of children with ADD/ADHD. *International Journal of Adolescent Medicine and Health.* 22:10;275–83.

Leisman G., Melillo R. 2010. R. Effects of motor sequence training on attentional performance in ADHD Children. *International Journal on Disability and Human Development.* 9(4);275–82.

Leisman G., Melillo R., Machado C. 2010. Functional disconnectivities in autistic spectrum individuals informs disorders of consciousness. *Medisur.* 8(1);76.

Leisman G., Melillo R. 2009. EEG coherence measures functional disconnectivities in autism. *Acta Paediatrica.* 98:460;1–292.

Leisman G., Melillo R. 2009. EEG coherence measures functional disconnectivities in autism. Paper presented at the 50th Annual Meeting of the European society for Paediatric Research, Hamburg, Germany, 9–12 October. Also published in *Acta Paediatrica.* 98:460; 1–292.

Leisman G., Melillo R. 2007. A call to arms: somatosensory perception, and action. *Behavioral and Brain Sciences.* 30:2;215.

Liu J. et al. 2014. Study on the association between diet, nutrients and attention deficit hyperactivity disorder among children in Shanghai, Kunshan, Wuxi three kindergarten. *Journal of Hygiene Research.* March;43(2):235–39.

Lockner D.W., Crowe T.K., Skipper B.J. 2008. Dietary intake and parents' perception of mealtime behaviors in preschool-age children with autism spectrum disorder and in typically developing children. *Journal of the American Dietetic Association.* Aug.;108(8):1360–63.

Lohmann C. 2009. Calcium signaling and the development of specific neuronal connections. *Progress In Brain Research.* 175:443–52.

Machado C., Estevez M., Leisman G., Melillo R. et al. 2015. EEG coherence assessment of autistic children in three different experimental conditions. *Journal of Autism and Developmental Disorders.* 45:406–24. doi: 10.1007/s10803-013-1909-5.

Machado C., Estevez M., Melillo R., Leisman G. et al. 2013. Quantitative resting EEG in the autistic spectrum disorder. *International Journal of Child Health and Human Development.* 6(4):511.

Machado C., Estevez M., Leisman G., Melillo R., Machado A., Hernanandez-Cruz A., Arias A., Rodriguez-Rojas R., Carballo M. 2013. Exploration of resting brain connectivity using linear coherence measures in the autistic spectrum disorder. *Chronic Disease and Disability in Childhood.* Haupaugue, NY: Nova Scientific, p. 149.

Machado C., Estevez M., Melillo R., Leisman G., Carrick R., Machado A., Hernandez-Cruz A., Arias A., Rodriguez-Rojas R., Carballo M. 2013. Quantitative resting EEG in the autistic spectrum disorder. *Chronic Disease and Disability in Childhood.* Haupaugue, NY: Nova Scientific, p. 150.

Machado C., Rodríguez R., Estevez M., Leisman G., Chinchilla M., Melillo R. 2015. Electrophysiologic and fMRI anatomic and functional connectivity relationships in autistic children during three different experimental conditions. *Brain Connectivity.* 2015. Sept. 18 [Epub ahead of print]

Melillo R., Leisman G. 2015. Functional Brain Imbalance and Autism Spectrum Disorder. Olfman, S. (ed.) *The Science and Pseudoscience of Children's Mental Illness: Cutting Edge Research and Treatment. Childhood In America Book Series.* Santa Barbara, CA: Praeger.

Melillo R., Leisman G. 2010. *Neurobehavioral Disorders of Childhood: An Evolutionary Perspective.* New York, NY: Springer Science, 2010.

Melillo R.M., Leisman G. 2009. Autism spectrum disorder as functional disconnection syndrome. *Reviews in the Neurosciences.* 20:2;111–32.

Melillo R.M., Leisman G. 2007. *Neurobehavioral Disorders of Childhood: An Evolutionary Perspective.* Seoul, Korea: G. Panmun Book Co., Ltd, 2007.

Mennella J.A., Johnson A., Beauchamp G.J. 1995. Garlic ingestion by pregnant women alters the odor of amniotic fluid. *Chemical Senses.* April;20(2):207–9.

Naushad S.M. et al. 2013. Autistic children exhibit distinct plasma amino acid profile. *Indian Journal of Biochemistry & Biophysics.* Oct.;50(5):474–78.

Ogden C.L. et al. 2002. Prevalence and trends in overweight among US children and adolescents, 1999–2000. *JAMA.* Oct. 9;288(14):1728–32.

Olson C.R., Mello C.V. 2010. Significance of vitamin A to brain function, behavior and learning. *Molecular Nutrition & Food Research.* April;54(4):489–95.

Parr J. 2010. Autism. *Clinical Evidence (Online).* Jan.7;pii:0322.

Raymond L., Deth R.C., Ralston N.V. 2014. Potential role of selenoenzymes and antioxidant metabolism in relation to autism etiology and pathology. *Autism research and treatment.* March 5 Epub.

Rimland B. 1988. Controversies in the treatment of autistic children: vitamin and drug therapy. *Journal of Child Neurology.* 3 Suppl:S68–72.

Rodriguez-Rojas R., Leisman G., Melillo R. et al. 2013. Anatomical and topological connectivity reveal different attributes of disrupted small-world networks in autistic children. *International Journal of Child Health and Human Development.* 6(4):551.

Savage J.S., Fisher J.O., Birch L.L. 2007. Parental influence on eating behavior: conception to adolescence. *Journal of Law, Medicine & Ethics.* Spring;35(1):22–34.

Schlief M.L. et al. 2006. Role of the Menkes copper-transporting ATPase in NMDA receptor-mediated neuronal toxicity. *Proceedings of the National Academy of Science.* Oct. 3;103(40):14919–24.

Stevens L. et al. 2003. EFA supplementation in children with inattention, hyperactivity, and other disruptive behaviors. *Lipids.* Oct.;38(10):1007–21.

INDEX

acorn squash: Stuffed Acorn Squash,
158–59
Adderal, 7–8
addiction to foods, 16–17, 24, 46
adolescence, 8, 71–72
aggressive behavior, 16
agricultural system, 8–9
allergies, 104
All-Natural Homemade Ketchup, 143–44
almond butter
Almond-Peanut Butter Protein Balls,
203–4
Swiss Almond-Chocolate Smoothie, 213
almonds
Chocolate-Almond Smoothie, 128
Dr Ed's Almond Cereal, 122–23
alpha lipoic acid, 114–15
Amasai cultured dairy yogurt, 212
American Academy of Pediatrics, 13, 60
American Heart Association, 87
amino acids, 90
Anderson, Linda, 178
antibiotics, 9, 45, 67–68
antioxidants, 90, 94, 106, 110–11
appetite, 7–8, 42, 99
apples
Apple Carrot Cake, 191–92
Donna's Gluten-Free Pie Crust and Pie
Fillings, 198–200
and 10 Most Wanted List, 46
Art Café recipes
Banana Bread, 194–95
Blueberry Muffins, 195–96
Gluten-Free Bread, 183–84
Gluten-Free Chocolate-Chip Cookies,
197–98
art with food, 80

arugula, 165
asparagus: Grilled Asparagus, 178–79
Asperger's syndrome, xix, 5, 76
attention, 10, 28, 37
attention deficit/hyperactive disorder
(ADHD)
and alpha lipoic acid, 114
and brain balance approach, 11–12
diagnosis of, xviii
and elimination diet, 91
and essential fatty acids, 113
and functional disconnection syndrome, 3
and genetics, xix
and inflammatory responses, 16
and magnesium, 108
medications for, 7–8
and nutritional deficiencies, 90, 91, 108
and nutritional supplements, 91
and oral-motor weakness, 26
relationship of diet to, 9
as right-brain deficiency, xxi, 5
and selenium, 110
and sugar consumption, 9
and trying new foods, 34
and vitamin C, 103
auditory sense, 4, 6, 37
authoritative vs. authoritarian parenting, 73
Autism (Melillo), xix, 49, 105
autism and autism spectrum
and antioxidants, 90
and calcium, 107
and Coenzyme Q10, 115–16
and copper, 110
diagnosis of, xviii
and folate/folic acid, 99, 102
food issues associated with, xxii
and functional disconnection syndrome, 3

autism and autism spectrum (*cont.*)
    and genetics, xix, 49
    and homocysteine, 96
    and immature gastrointestinal systems,
        10
    and leaky gut syndrome, 13
    and magnesium, 108
    and nutritional deficiencies, 90, 91, 99,
        107, 108
    and omega-3 fatty acids, 113
    and oral-motor weakness, 26
    and overactive sympathetic nervous
        system, 10
    perceived as untreatable, xviii
    relationship of diet to, 9
    as right-brain deficiency, xxi, 5
    and sensory processing imbalances, 28
    and vitamin A, 95
    and vitamin B-6, 98, 99
    and vitamin B-12, 96–97, 99
    and vitamin C, 104
    and vitamin D, 105
    and zinc, 109, 110
Autism Research Institute, 91
Autumn Beauty Fruit Salad, 175–76
avocados
    Avocado Smoothie, 212
    Avocado-Spinach Quinoa, 140–41
    Mango-Avocado Salsa, 146–47

bacteria of the gut (microbiota), 13, 29–30
bagels, gluten-free, 154
baked goods, 181–200
    about, 181–82
    Apple Carrot Cake, 191–92
    Art Café Banana Bread, 194–95
    Art Café Blueberry Muffins, 195–96
    Art Café Gluten-Free Chocolate-Chip
        Cookies, 197–98
    Art Café's Gluten-Free Bread, 183–84
    Basic All-Occasion Cake, 185–86
    Cheesy Drop Rolls, 186–87
    Dark Chocolate Brownies, 193–94
    Donna's Gluten-Free Pie Crust and Pie
        Fillings, 198–200
    and egg substitutes, 184–85
    and gluten-free flours, 181–82, 188–89
    Graham Cracker Cookies, 196–97
    Potato Pizza Crust, 189–90

So-Easy Chocolate Brownies, 192–93
    Tony's Pizza Dough, 190–91
    See also breads
Baked Kale Chips, 210–11
baker's yeast, 45
bananas
    Art Café Banana Bread, 194–95
    Banana-Berry Cereal, 125
    Banana Cream Smoothie, 213
    Cherry-Banana Buckwheat Pudding,
        126–27
    Oatmeal Chocolate-Chip Cookies,
        207–8
    Strawberry-Banana Smoothie, 127–28
barley, 44
Basic All-Occasion Cake, 185–86
BBQ sauce recipe, 144–45
beans, 45, 88
bedwetting, 16
beef
    Dr. Dave's Molé Chili, 160–61
    Stuffed Red Bell Peppers, 159–60
beets: Golden Beet Salad, 169–70
behavioral issues
    and apples, 46
    and calcium, 107
    and elimination diet, 50
    and food sensitivities, 48, 50, 52
    and ignoring inappropriate behaviors,
        78–79
    and inflammatory responses, 16
    and rewarding behaviors, 77–78, 79
    and sugar consumption, 65
    and vitamin E, 106
bell peppers
    Grilled Veggie Salad, 173–74
    Stuffed Red Bell Peppers, 159–60
berries: Banana-Berry Cereal, 125
beta-carotene, 95
A Better Mac and Cheese, 141–42
biotin, 91, 102–3
Birthday Blueberry Muffins, 131
black beans: Sweet Potato/Black Bean Bur-
    ritos in Collard Wraps, 161–62
bloating, 67
blood sugar regulation, 65–67
blueberries
    Art Café Blueberry Muffins, 195–96
    Birthday Blueberry Muffins, 131

bok choy, 165
bottles, difficulties with, 31
bowel obstruction, 42
brain
  and B vitamins, 99
  effect of poor diet on, 6–7
  foggy or sluggish, 16, 18
  fuel of, 7, 89
  as governor of organ systems, 4–5
  nutritional needs of, 6, 89–93, 94–116
  stimulation needs of, 7, 89
Brain Balance Achievement Centers, xvii, xxiii
breading foods, 85–86
breads
  Art Café Banana Bread, 194–95
  Art Café Blueberry Muffins, 195–96
  Art Café's Gluten-Free Bread, 183–84
  Birthday Blueberry Muffins, 131
  Cheesy Drop Rolls, 186–87
  Cherry-Walnut Breakfast Loaf, 129
  and chronic yeast infections, 68
  gluten-free, 154
  and glycemic index (GI), 66
  Pumpkin Pie Muffins, 130
breakfast, 119–32
  Banana-Berry Cereal, 125
  Birthday Blueberry Muffins, 131
  Cherry-Banana Buckwheat Pudding, 126–27
  Cherry-Walnut Breakfast Loaf, 129
  Chocolate-Almond Smoothie, 128
  and clarified butter, 132
  Coconut Millet with Aromatic Spices, 124
  Dr Ed's Almond Cereal, 122–23
  Grain-Free Granola, 121–22
  importance of, 72, 119
  Instant Coconut-Cinnamon Breakfast Cereal, 120–21
  Pumpkin Pie Muffins, 130
  Rice Pudding, 127
  Slow Cooker Brown Rice Porridge, 123
  Strawberry-Banana Smoothie, 127–28
breast feeding, 31, 71
breathing, noisy, 42
brewer's yeast, 45, 68
broccoli: Pureed Vegetable Soup with a Kick, 133–34

Broiled Tandoori-Spiced Salmon with Avocado-Spinach Quinoa, 140–41
Brown, Zac, ix–xi, xiii–xvi, 11–12, 171
brownies
  Dark Chocolate Brownies, 193–94
  So-Easy Chocolate Brownies, 192–93
brown rice: Slow Cooker Brown Rice Porridge, 123
buckwheat: Cherry-Banana Buckwheat Pudding, 126–27
bulk bins in supermarkets, 125
burritos: Sweet Potato/Black Bean Burritos in Collard Wraps, 161–62
butter
  clarifying, 132
  substitutions for, 153
butternut squash
  Moroccan Chicken Salad, 151–52
  Pureed Vegetable Soup with a Kick, 133–34
B vitamins
  and ADHD, 91
  biotin, 102–3
  as brain food, 99
  deficiencies in, 42
  vitamin B-1 (thiamine), 90, 91, 98–99
  vitamin B-3 (niacin), 90, 91, 100
  vitamin B-5 (pantothenic acid), 91, 100–101
  vitamin B-6 (pyridoxine), 90, 97–98, 99
  vitamin B-12, 13, 96–97, 99

cabbage
  Pocketknife Coleslaw, 171–72
  Turkey, Cabbage, and Carrots over Rice, 154
Cajun Red Potato Fries, 166
cakes
  Apple Carrot Cake, 191–92
  Basic All-Occasion Cake, 185–86
calcium
  and ADHD, 91
  and autism, 90
  and brain health, 107
Camp Southern Ground, x, xiii–xvi, 11
Candida albicans, 67
candy, 54
Candy-Cane Carrots, 177–78
canned foods, 88

canola oil, 88
carbohydrates, 9, 90, 91
Carlson, Lisa, 136, 150
carrots
    Apple Carrot Cake, 191–92
    Candy-Cane Carrots, 177–78
    Golden Beet Salad, 169–70
    Pureed Vegetable Soup with a Kick,
        133–34
    Turkey, Cabbage, and Carrots over Rice,
        154
casein
    and clarified butter, 132
    and *Disconnected Kids* recipes, 119
    and elimination diet, 52
    and 10 Most Wanted List, 44–45
cattle, 9
Cave Man nutrition bars, 154
celiac disease, 44
central auditory processing disorder, 6
cereals
    Banana-Berry Cereal, 125
    Dr Ed's Almond Cereal, 122–23
    Instant Coconut-Cinnamon Breakfast
        Cereal, 120–21
cheese
    and chronic yeast infections, 68
    and elimination diet, 45, 54
cheese alternatives
    A Better Mac and Cheese, 141–42
    Cheesy Drop Rolls, 186–87
    Cheesy Kale Chips, 211–12
    Linguine Alfredo, 156
    suggestions for, 153
cherries
    Cherry-Banana Buckwheat Pudding,
        126–27
    Cherry-Coconut Power Bars, 202–3
    Cherry-Walnut Breakfast Loaf, 129
chia seeds: Instant Coconut-Cinnamon
    Breakfast Cereal, 120–21
chicken
    Chicken-Quinoa Soup, 135–36
    Chicken-Rice Soup, 135
    Coconut-Crusted Chicken Fingers,
        145–46
    Coconut Curry Soup, 136–37
    Crispy Pan-Fried Chicken, 149
    Fried Chicken Tenders, 147–49

    Garbanzo Bean Fried Chicken, 142–43
    Lemon-Pepper Chicken-on-a-Stick,
        139–40
    Moroccan Chicken Salad, 151–52
chickpeas
    digestibility of, 46
    and garbanzo flour recipes, 142–43,
        155–56
    Pureed Vegetable Soup with a Kick,
        133–34
chili: Dr. Dave's Molé Chili, 160–61
chocolate
    Art Café Gluten-Free Chocolate-Chip
        Cookies, 197–98
    Chocolate-Almond Smoothie, 128
    Chocolate-Chip Peanut Butter Crisps,
        206
    Chocolate-Peanut Butter Swirl Cups,
        207
    Dark Chocolate Brownies, 193–94
    Oatmeal Chocolate-Chip Cookies,
        207–8
    Peanut Butter Chocolate-Chip Cookie
        Balls, 204–5
    So-Easy Chocolate Brownies, 192–93
    Swiss Almond-Chocolate Smoothie, 213
choking, 25, 42
Chunky Tomato Salsa, 147
cinnamon
    Cinnamon-Spiced Sweet Potato, 167–68
    Instant Coconut-Cinnamon Breakfast
        Cereal, 120–21
citrus, 47–48, 104
clarified butter, 132
coconut
    Cherry-Coconut Power Bars, 202–3
    Coconut-Crusted Chicken Fingers,
        145–46
    Coconut Curry Soup, 136–37
    Coconut Millet with Aromatic Spices,
        124
    Coconut Nut Balls, 209
    Dr Ed's Almond Cereal, 122–23
    Grain-Free Granola, 121–22
    Instant Coconut-Cinnamon Breakfast
        Cereal, 120–21
    and sulfites, 203
coconut milk
    Power Popsicles, 208

Pumpkin-Coconut Rice Pudding, 209–10
recommendations for, 153
Coenzyme Q10 (CoQ10), 115–16
coleslaw recipe: Pocketknife Coleslaw, 171–72
colic, 42
collard greens
nutritional benefits of, 165
Sweet Potato/Black Bean Burritos in Collard Wraps, 161–62
colors, 38–39
complexion, pale or sallow, 16
computers and screens, 7–8
concentration, 10, 16, 30
condiments
Chunky Tomato Salsa, 147
and food chaining process, 86
Mango-Avocado Salsa, 146–47
Stacey's All-Natural Homemade Ketchup, 143–44
Stacey's Caribbean-Style BBQ Sauce, 144–45
conduct disorder, 5, 9
constipation
and chronic yeast infections, 67
and leaky gut syndrome, 13
and manganese, 111
cookies
Art Café Gluten-Free Chocolate-Chip Cookies, 197–98
Chocolate-Chip Peanut Butter Crisps, 206
Graham Cracker Cookies, 196–97
Oatmeal Chocolate-Chip Cookies, 207–8
Peanut Butter Chocolate-Chip Cookie Balls, 204–5
cooking with children, 81
copper, 110
corn, 47, 64
corn syrup, 68
cortisol, 8, 65
coughing when eating, 25, 42
Cranberry Confetti Wild Rice, 171
cravings, 17, 46
cream, substitutes for, 153
Crispy Pan-Fried Chicken, 149
cucumbers

Cucumber Salad, 175
Golden Beet Salad, 169–70
curry: Coconut Curry Soup, 136–37
cytokines, 15

Daily Values (DV), 96
dairy
and addictions to foods, 17
avoiding, 89
and elimination diet, 52–53, 56
and food labels, 62–63
substitutions for, 153
and 10 Most Wanted List, 44–45
Daiya brand cheese alternatives
A Better Mac and Cheese, 141–42
Linguine Alfredo, 156
as recommended brand, 153
Dark Chocolate Brownies, 193–94
Davidson, Kristen, 120, 161
Davis, T. William, 66
Deceptively Delicious (Seinfeld), 85
dehydration, 60
depression, 54
developmental delays, xx, 29
developmental milestones, 19–22
diabetes, 6
diarrhea, 13, 42, 67
digestive system
and chronic yeast infections, 67
and digestive enzymes, 115
and food sensitivities, 15
immature, xxi–xxii, 10
and nutritional malabsorption, 90
and pesticides, 87
primary dysfunctions in, 10
and underresponsive sensory systems, 27
See also leaky gut syndrome
dinner recipes, 139–63
A Better Mac and Cheese, 141–42
Broiled Tandoori-Spiced Salmon with Avocado-Spinach Quinoa, 140–41
Coconut-Crusted Chicken Fingers, 145–46
Crispy Pan-Fried Chicken, 149
Dr. Dave's Molé Chili, 160–61
Fried Chicken Tenders, 147–49
Garbanzo Bean Fried Chicken, 142–43
Garbanzo Bean Fried Shrimp, 155–56
Grub Worms and Dirt Bombs, 157–58

dinner recipes (*cont.*)
  Lemon-Pepper Chicken-on-a-Stick,
    139–40
  Linguine Alfredo, 156
  Moroccan Chicken Salad, 151–52
  Slow-Cooker Pork Chops, 155
  Spaghetti and Spanish Meatballs, 158
  Stuffed Acorn Squash, 158–59
  Stuffed Red Bell Peppers, 159–60
  Sweet Potato/Black Bean Burritos in
    Collard Wraps, 161–62
  Taco Seasoning, 163
  Turkey, Cabbage, and Carrots over Rice,
    154
  Turkey Potpie, 152–53
Disconnected Kids (Melillo)
  assessments in, 20
  on autism treatment, xviii
  on Functional Disconnection Syndrome,
    xvii
  and nutritional needs of kids, 89
  on sensory issues, 33, 37, 38, 39
Dr. Dave's Molé Chili, 160–61
Dr. Ed's Almond Cereal, 122–23
Donna's Gluten-Free Pie Crust and Pie
    Fillings, 198–200
dosages of nutrients, 92, 96
drooling, 26, 28
dyscalculia, 6
dyslexia, xviii, xix, 3, 6
dyspraxia, 6

ear infections, 67
Earth Balance butter substitute, 153
eating out, 73
eggs
  and food labels, 63–64
  substitutions for, 184–85
  and 10 Most Wanted List, 45
Elgar, Frank, 72
elimination diet
  about, 43
  and ADHD, 91
  and rotation diet, 58–60
  Step 1: documentation, 50–51
  Step 2: looking for patterns, 51–52
  Step 3: eliminating suspect foods, 52–55
  Step 4: reintroducing foods, 56–57
  Step 5: drawing conclusions, 57–58

  and ten common food culprits, 44–48
  and testing for IgG food intolerance, 57
  and withdrawal symptoms, 54
emotional issues, 16
epigenetic effects, xx–xxi, 49
essential fatty acids, 90, 91, 113–15
estrogen levels, 47
exercise, 70
eyes, puffiness or dark circles under, 16

face, food on, 35–36
facial muscles, weak, 25
family dinners, 71–72
family history of food sensitivity, 49–50
farming, conventional, 8–9
fast food, 10, 54
fatigue, 16, 96
fats, 9, 91
fatty acids, 90, 91, 113–15
fermented foods, 68
fiber, 91
Finucan, Ed, 121
fish, 87, 90, 95
fish oil supplementation, 91
flavors, 70, 71, 74, 80
flax meal
  Instant Coconut-Cinnamon Breakfast
    Cereal, 120–21
  Pumpkin Pie Muffins, 130
flours, gluten-free, 181–82, 188–89
flour substitutes, 154
fluorescent lighting, 39
focus, 10, 16, 30
folate and folic acid, 13, 90
food additives, 54
food aversion, 31
food chaining, 82–86
food labels, 62–65
food sensitivities, 14–17
  and addictions to foods, 16–17
  and behavioral symptoms, 48, 50, 52
  and epigenetics, 49
  and food allergies, 14, 17, 48
  and food labels, 62–65
  and high-glycemic foods, 67
  and IgG food intolerance testing, 57
  and inflammation, 19
  and leaky gut syndrome, 15
  and right-brain deficiencies, 17, 52

symptoms of, 16
ten common culprits, 44–48
See also elimination diet
food supply issues, 8–9
Fried Chicken Tenders, 147–49
fries
    Cajun Red Potato Fries, 166
    Sweet Potato Fries, 168–69
frozen foods, 87, 165
fruits
    Autumn Beauty Fruit Salad, 175–76
    canned, 88
    consumption of, in U.S., 165
    dried fruits, 68
    fruit juice, 60
    guidelines for, 87
    Hawaiian Fruit Salad, 176–77
    and rotation diet, 60
fudge: Peanut Butter Fudge, 205–6
Fugo, Jennifer, xxiv, 123, 125, 149, 173
Functional Disconnection Syndrome (FDS)
    and Brain Balance approach, xix–xx
    cause of, xvii
    and digestive enzymes, 115
    disorders commonly associated with, 3
    and epigenetic effects, xx–xxi
    food issues associated with, xxii
    and homocysteine, 96, 101
    and manganese, 111
    and molybdenum, 112
    and nutritional deficiencies, 90
    and poor diet, 92
functional medicine field, 18
functional neurology field, 18, 92
functional nutrition, 92
fungicides, 9

Gadbois, Stacey
    breakfast recipes of, 131
    dinner recipes of, 142, 143, 154, 155, 158,
        159
    snack recipes of, 201, 205, 207, 209
    vegetable recipes of, 167
gagging, 42
games with foods, 81
garbanzo beans (chickpeas)
    digestibility of, 46
    Pureed Vegetable Soup with a Kick,
        133–34

garbanzo flour
    Garbanzo Bean Fried Chicken, 142–43
    Garbanzo Bean Fried Shrimp, 155–56
genetically modified organisms (GMO), 47
genetics and gene expression
    and autism, xix, 49
    and developmental delays, xx
    environmental influences on, xxi, 49–50
    and nutrients, 13, 102, 103
Gentile, David A., 160, 170
ghee, 132
glucose, 6, 7, 65–66
gluten
    avoiding, 87, 89
    and bulk bins, 125
    and *Disconnected Kids* recipes, 119, 120
    and elimination diet, 52
    gluten-free flours, 181–82, 188–89
    and grains, 125
    and store-bought gluten-free options, 154
    and 10 Most Wanted List, 44
    See also baked goods
glycemic index (GI), 66–67
Golden Beet Salad with Rainbow Carrots,
        Cucumber, and Nutty Herb Vinai-
        grette, 169–70
Gordon-Teixeira, Donna, xxiv, 181–82
    baked goods recipes of, 185–87, 192–96,
        197–99
    dinner recipes of, 141, 189–90
    egg replacer of, 184–85
    gluten-free flour blend of, 182, 188–89
Graham Cracker Cookies, 196–97
granola
    Grain-Free Granola, 121–22
    Healthier Granola Bars, 201–2
green, calming effect of, 38
Green Beans with Honey, 178
greens, leafy
    Baked Kale Chips, 210–11
    benefits of, 95, 165
    Cheesy Kale Chips, 211–12
    Hawaiian Fruit Salad, 176–77
    Pureed Vegetable Soup with a Kick,
        133–34
    South-of-the-Border Salad, 170
    Summer Festival Salad, 174–75
Grilled Asparagus, 178–79
Grilled Veggie Salad, 173–74

Grub Worms and Dirt Bombs, 157–58
guar gum, 182
gulping sounds, 25, 26, 31
gurgling while eating, 31
gut–brain axis, 30

Hamlin, Rusty
    dinner recipes of, 139
    vegetable recipes of, 166, 169, 171, 174,
        175, 177, 178
hands-on with foods, 80
Hawaiian Fruit Salad, 176–77
headaches, 16
Healthier Granola Bars, 201–2
heartburn, 42
heart disease, 6
herbicides, 9
"hiding" nutrition in foods, 85
hippocampus, 105
hives, 42
homocysteine, 96, 98, 101
honey
    and chronic yeast infections, 68
    Green Beans with Honey, 178
hormones, 4, 9, 65
hydration, 60
hyperactivity
    and alpha lipoic acid, 114
    and apples, 46
    and food sensitivities, 16
    and high-glycemic foods, 66
    and magnesium, 108
    and processed foods, 90
hyper/hypoglycemia, 66

identification of foods, 30
IgG food intolerance testing, 57
immune systems
    and chronic inflammation, 18–19
    and food sensitivities, 15, 17
    and functional disconnection syndrome, 4
    and magnesium, 108
    and organic foods, 87
    of problem feeders, 4
    and Strawberry-Banana Smoothie, 128
    and vitamin B-5, 100
immunoglobulin G (IgG), 57
Importance of Family Dinners VII (report),
    72

impulsive actions, 16
inflammation
    behavioral/emotional symptoms of,
        15–16
    effects of, 18–19
    and food sensitivities, 15, 17
    and functional disconnection syndrome,
        4
    and leaky gut syndrome, 17
    and magnesium, 108
    and molybdenum, 112
ingredients, guidelines for, 88
Instant Coconut-Cinnamon Breakfast
    Cereal, 120–21
insulin, 65–66
intestines
    bacteria in, 29–30
    dysfunctions in, 10
    and inflammation, 18, 19
iron, 90, 91
irritability
    and elimination diet, 54
    and food sensitivities, 16
    and high-glycemic foods, 66
    and magnesium, 108

Jackson, Rebecca, 130, 133, 134, 151, 158
Josh Prichard's Kickin' Vegan Potato Salad,
    166–67
Journal of the American Dietetic Association,
    95
junk foods, 54, 78, 90

kale
    Baked Kale Chips, 210–11
    Cheesy Kale Chips, 211–12
    Pureed Vegetable Soup with a Kick,
        133–34
ketchup, 143–44
Kind nutrition bars, 154
kiwis
    Autumn Beauty Fruit Salad, 175–76
    Hawaiian Fruit Salad, 176–77
Korth, Christie, xxiv
    breakfast recipes of, 124, 126, 127
    dinner recipes of, 152, 157
    fruit recipes of, 176
    soup recipes of, 135
    on sulfites in coconuts, 203

on trying new foods, 34–35
vegetable recipes of, 172
Kral, Tanja V. E., 74

lactobacillus acidophilus, 68
lactobacillus plantarum, 68
lactose intolerance, 45
language disorders, 6
Lapine, Missy, 85
LäraBars, 154
Law of Attraction, 82
lead, 19
leafy greens
    Baked Kale Chips, 210–11
    benefits of, 95, 165
    Cheesy Kale Chips, 211–12
    Hawaiian Fruit Salad, 176–77
    Pureed Vegetable Soup with a Kick,
        133–34
    South-of-the-Border Salad, 170
    Summer Festival Salad, 174–75
leaky gut syndrome
    and addictions to foods, 16–17
    and citrus, 47
    and digestive enzymes, 115
    and dysfunctions in digestive system, 10
    and eggs, 45
    and food sensitivities, 15
    and gluten, 44
    and legumes, 45
    and nutritional deficiencies, xxi–xxii,
        13–14, 92
    and nutritional malabsorption, 90
    and tomatoes, 46
learning disabilities
    diagnosis of, xviii
    and food sensitivities, 16
    and functional disconnection syndrome, 3
    as left-brain deficiency, 6
    and nutritional supplements, 91
    and oral-motor weakness, 26
    as right-brain deficiency, 5
left-brain imbalance, 5, 6, 56, 67
legs, pain in, 16
legumes, 45
Lemon-Pepper Chicken-on-a-Stick,
    139–40
lethargy, 54, 97
lighting, 37, 39

limited diet, consequences of, 29–30
Linguine Alfredo, 156
Lisa's Multipurpose Chicken, 136, 150
livestock, 9
Lowenthal, Heather, 168, 191, 196–97

mac-and-cheese recipe, 141–42
magnesium, 90, 91, 98, 108
manganese, 111
mangos
    Hawaiian Fruit Salad, 176–77
    Mango-Avocado Salsa, 146–47
maple syrup, 68
McGregor, Hadley, 129, 156
mealtime, sitting through, 39–40
meats
    and food chaining process, 86
    guidelines for, 87
    and niacin, 100
    processed, 90
    and vitamin B-5, 101
medications
    for ADHD, 7–8
    antibiotics, 9, 45, 67–68
    and Brain Balance approach, xviii
melatonin, 8
Melillo, Susan, 128
Melillo 7-Day Challenge, 20, 219–20
memory, 30
mental health, 72
mercury, 19
microbiota, 13, 29–30
migraines, 16
milk
    alternatives to, 87
    and elimination diet, 52–53, 56
    and 10 Most Wanted List, 44–45
millet: Coconut Millet with Aromatic
        Spices, 124
minerals, 90
modeling healthy eating, 69–71, 74
molé chili recipe, 160–61
molybdenum, 112–13
moods, 30
Moroccan Chicken Salad, 151–52
Most Wanted List, 44–48, 65
motor planning problems, 6
muffins
    Art Café Blueberry Muffins, 195–96

muffins (*cont.*)
  Birthday Blueberry Muffins, 131
  Pumpkin Pie Muffins, 130
Multipurpose Chicken, 136, 150
multivitamins, 92
muscle pain, 16
mushrooms
  Stuffed Red Bell Peppers, 159–60
  Summer Festival Salad, 174–75

Namaste Foods Gluten-Free Perfect Flour
  Blend, 154
National Academy of Sciences, 8
National Center on Addiction and Substance Abuse, 72
neophobia, 75
new foods
  and food chaining process, 82–86
  multiple exposures to, 74, 75
  procedure for introducing, 34–35
  refusal of, 24, 75
niacin (vitamin B-3), 90, 91, 100
noisy environments, 37–38
noses (stuffy, itchy, runny), 16
nut butters, 88
Nutrients, 90
nutrition bars, 154
nutritionists, 18
nuts
  Cheesy Kale Chips, 211–12
  Coconut Nut Balls, 209
  and rotation diet, 60

oats
  Cherry-Coconut Power Bars, 202–3
  Healthier Granola Bars, 201–2
  Oatmeal Chocolate-Chip Cookies,
    207–8
obesity, 6, 69, 74
obsessive-compulsive disorder (OCD), 5,
  34
olfactory issues. *See* smell, sense of
olive oil, 88
omega-3 fatty acids, 91, 113–14
omega-6 fatty acids, 91
opiates, 17
oppositional defiant disorder (ODD), xviii,
  xix, xxi
oral-motor skills, 25–26

orange juice, 47–48
organic foods, 87, 120
overeating, 27, 78
oxidative stress, 90, 106, 115
oxygen, 7

packaged foods, 47, 62, 88
pain, 16
pantothenic acid (vitamin B-5), 90, 91,
  100–101
papayas
  Hawaiian Fruit Salad, 176–77
  Papaya Smoothie, 214
parents
  authoritative vs. authoritarian, 73
  and breakfast, 72
  and child-friendly meals, 77
  and family dinners, 71–72
  and food choices during pregnancy, 71
  gatekeeper role of, 70
  and ignoring inappropriate behaviors,
    78–79
  and meals away from home, 73
  and rewarding behaviors, 77–78, 79
  as role models, 69–71, 74
  and routine meal times, 78
  serving different meals to kids, 77
  and tactics for managing mealtimes, 82
  willingness of, to be uncomfortable,
    74–75
pasta
  addiction to, 16–17
  A Better Mac and Cheese, 141–42
  Grub Worms and Dirt Bombs, 157–58
  Linguine Alfredo, 156
  Spaghetti and Spanish Meatballs, 158
Peaches-and-Cream Smoothie, 214
peanut butter
  Almond-Peanut Butter Protein Balls,
    203–4
  Chocolate-Chip Peanut Butter Crisps,
    206
  Chocolate-Peanut Butter Swirl Cups,
    207
  guidelines for, 46
  Healthier Granola Bars, 201–2
  Peanut Butter Chocolate-Chip Cookie
    Balls, 204–5
  Peanut Butter Fudge, 205–6

peas, 45
pecans: Grain-Free Granola, 121–22
Pediatrics, 90
peristalsis, 13
persimmons: Autumn Beauty Fruit Salad,
175–76
pervasive developmental disorder (PDD),
5, 98
pesticides, 8–9, 19, 87
physical activity, 7–8, 70
phytoestrogens, 47
picky eaters
and brain imbalance, 25
characteristics of, 23–24
and child-friendly meals, 77
and food aversion, 31
and food chaining process, 82–86
pie: Donna's Gluten-Free Pie Crust and Pie
Fillings, 198–200
Piña Colada Smoothie, 215
pizzas
Potato Pizza Crust, 189–90
Tony's Pizza Dough, 190–91
playtime with foods, 81
Pocketknife Coleslaw, 171–72
pollution, 9
pomegranate seeds: Autumn Beauty Fruit
Salad, 175–76
popsicle recipe, 208
pork
Slow-Cooker Pork Chops, 155
Spaghetti and Spanish Meatballs, 158
porridge: Slow Cooker Brown Rice Porridge, 123
portion sizes, 38, 87
Portman, Connie, 120, 127, 145, 179
positive reinforcements, 79
potassium, 90, 112
potatoes
Cajun Red Potato Fries, 166
Josh Prichard's Kickin' Vegan Potato
Salad, 166–67
Potato Pizza Crust, 189–90
potpie recipe, 152–53
power bars recipe, 202–3
Power Popsicles, 208
praise, 79
pregnancy, food choices during, 71
prepackaged foods, 50

Prichard, Josh, 166
probiotics, 68
problem feeders
characteristics of, 24
faulty eating muscles of, 25–26
and food aversion, 31
picky eaters compared to, 23
prevalence of, 25
processed foods, 9, 10, 54, 62
Progress in Brain Research, 107
proprioception, sense of, 4, 39–40, 41
proteins
and ADHD, 91
Almond-Peanut Butter Protein Balls,
203–4
Cherry-Coconut Power Bars, 202–3
Power Popsicles, 208
and rotation diet, 60
puddings
Cherry-Banana Buckwheat Pudding,
126–27
Pumpkin-Coconut Rice Pudding,
209–10
Rice Pudding, 127
pumpkin
Donna's Gluten-Free Pie Crust and Pie
Fillings, 198–99
Pumpkin-Coconut Rice Pudding,
209–10
Pumpkin Pie Muffins, 130
pumpkin seeds: Grain-Free Granola,
121–22
Pureed Vegetable Soup with a Kick,
133–34

quinoa
Avocado-Spinach Quinoa, 140–41
Chicken-Quinoa Soup, 135–36
Stuffed Acorn Squash, 158–59
Toasted Quinoa Cran-Raisin Salad,
172–73

raisins: Toasted Quinoa Cran-Raisin Salad,
172–73
Recommended Dietary Allowance (RDA),
96
Reconnected Kids (Melillo), 52
refusing foods
and Coenzyme Q10 (CoQ10), 116

refusing foods (*cont.*)
    and oral-motor weakness, 26
    and repeated exposure, 35, 75
restaurants, 73
restrictions on foods, 78
retching, 42
rewarding behaviors, 77–78, 79
Rhoads, Casey, 204–5
rice
    Chicken-Rice Soup, 135
    Cranberry Confetti Wild Rice, 171
    Pumpkin-Coconut Rice Pudding,
        209–10
    Rice Pudding, 127
    Rice Stuffing, 179
    Slow Cooker Brown Rice Porridge, 123
    Turkey, Cabbage, and Carrots over Rice,
        154
right-brain deficiencies
    conditions associated with, 5–6
    and elimination diet, 56
    and food sensitivities, 17, 52
    and trying new foods, 34
    and weak vestibular system, 39–40
Ritalin, 7–8, 91
rolls: Cheesy Drop Rolls, 186–87
romaine, 165
rotation diet, 58–60
routine meal times, 78
Rubin, Jordan S., xxiv, 146, 212
rye, 44

salads
    Autumn Beauty Fruit Salad, 175–76
    Cucumber Salad, 175
    Golden Beet Salad, 169–70
    Grilled Veggie Salad, 173–74
    Hawaiian Fruit Salad, 176–77
    Josh Prichard's Kickin' Vegan Potato
        Salad, 166–67
    Moroccan Chicken Salad, 151–52
    South-of-the-Border Salad, 170
    Summer Festival Salad, 174–75
    Toasted Quinoa Cran-Raisin Salad,
        172–73
salicylates, 46
salmon
    Broiled Tandoori-Spiced Salmon, 140–41
    and shopping guidelines, 87

salsas, 146–47
salty snacks, 90
school lunchtimes, 37
Scire, Peter, xiii–xiv
screens, 7–8, 37, 74
seeds, 60
Seinfeld, Jessica, 85
selenium
    and ADHD, 90, 91
    and autism, 91
    and brain health, 106, 110–11
self-control, 75
senses and sensory issues, 26–29
    and appreciation of food, 3–4
    and brain balance approach, 11
    and food issues, xxii
    implications of, 30
    improvement of, 30, 32
    as left-brain deficiency, 6
    and motor skills, 28–29
    and problem feeders, 24–25
    and routine meal times, 78
    strategies for, 80–81
shopping, 81, 87–88, 125
shrimp: Garbanzo Bean Fried Shrimp,
    155–56
sleep
    disturbances in, 7, 16
    and elimination diet, 54, 56
    and inflammation, 16
    and magnesium, 108
    and oral-motor weakness, 26
    and snoring or mouth breathing, 26
    and vitamin E, 106
Slow-Cooker Brown Rice Porridge, 123
Slow-Cooker Pork Chops, 155
smell, sense of
    and appreciation of food, 3
    and sensory issues, 26, 27, 29, 32–33
smoothies, 212–15
    Avocado Smoothie, 212
    Banana Cream Smoothie, 213
    Chocolate-Almond Smoothie, 128
    Papaya Smoothie, 214
    Peaches-and-Cream Smoothie, 214
    Piña Colada Smoothie, 215
    Strawberry-Banana Smoothie, 127–28
    Total Omega Smoothie, 215
    Tropical Smoothie, 213–14

snacks, 201–15
  access to, 74
  Almond-Peanut Butter Protein Balls,
    203–4
  Baked Kale Chips, 210–11
  Cheesy Kale Chips, 211–12
  Cherry-Coconut Power Bars, 202–3
  Chocolate-Chip Peanut Butter Crisps,
    206
  Chocolate-Peanut Butter Swirl Cups,
    207
  Coconut Nut Balls, 209
  Healthier Granola Bars, 201–2
  Peanut Butter Chocolate-Chip Cookie
    Balls, 204–5
  Peanut Butter Fudge, 205–6
  Power Popsicles, 208
  Pumpkin-Coconut Rice Pudding,
    209–10
  salty, 90
The Sneaky Chef (Lapine), 85
So Delicious dairy substitute, 153
So-Easy Chocolate Brownies, 192–93
soft drinks, 54
soups, 133–37
  Chicken-Quinoa Soup, 135–36
  Chicken-Rice Soup, 135
  Coconut Curry Soup, 136–37
  as pantry staple, 88
  Pureed Vegetable Soup with a Kick,
    133–34
  Thai Sweet-Potato Soup, 134–35
  and vegetable consumption, 165
South-of-the-Border Salad, 170
soy
  as common ingredient, 47, 50
  and food labels, 64–65
  and 10 Most Wanted List, 46–47
spaghetti and meatballs recipes
  Grub Worms and Dirt Bombs, 157–58
  Spaghetti and Spanish Meatballs, 158
speech therapists, 26
spicy foods, 27
spilling foods and drinks, 28
spinach: Avocado-Spinach Quinoa, 140–41
spinal gallant reflex, 40, 41
spitting up, 42
squash
  Grilled Veggie Salad, 173–74

Moroccan Chicken Salad, 151–52
Pureed Vegetable Soup with a Kick,
    133–34
Stuffed Acorn Squash, 158–59
squirming, 41
Stacey's All-Natural Homemade Ketchup,
    143–44
Stacey's Caribbean-Style BBQ Sauce,
    144–45
stimulants, 7–8
stomach, 10
Strawberry-Banana Smoothie, 127–28
stress response, 65–66
Stuffed Acorn Squash, 158–59
Stuffed Red Bell Peppers, 159–60
stuffing: Rice Stuffing, 179
substitutions for common foods, 153–54
sugar
  and ADHD, 9
  and blood sugar regulation, 65–67
  and chronic yeast infections, 67, 68
  cravings for, 67
  guidelines for, 87, 89
  negative effects of, 6
  occasional consumption of, 201
  in processed foods, 9
  and underdeveloped taste perception, 29
Summer Festival Salad, 174–75
sunflower seeds: Grain-Free Granola,
    121–22
swallowing, difficulty with, 42
Swarthout, Janeil, 125, 175–76, 211–12
sweet potatoes
  Cinnamon-Spiced Sweet Potato, 167–68
  Sweet Potato/Black Bean Burritos in
    Collard Wraps, 161–62
  Sweet Potato Fries, 168–69
  Thai Sweet-Potato Soup, 134–35
Swiss Almond-Chocolate Smoothie, 213
Swiss chard, 165
sympathetic nervous system, 10, 15

table manners, 39–40
table settings, 38
Taco Seasoning, 163
Talking Stick Method, 38
taste, sense of, 4, 26
teenagers, 71–72
textures of foods, 29, 36–37, 80

Thai Sweet-Potato Soup, 134–35
thiamine (vitamin B-1), 90, 91, 98–99
Toasted Quinoa Cran-Raisin Salad, 172–73
tomatoes
  Chunky Tomato Salsa, 147
  Stacey's All-Natural Homemade Ketch-
    up, 143–44
  Summer Festival Salad, 174–75
  and 10 Most Wanted List, 46
Tony's Pizza Dough, 190–91
Total Omega Smoothie, 215
touch and hyperactive tactile systems
  aversion to touching foods, 4, 24, 35–36
  strategies for, 36–37, 80
Tourette's syndrome, xxi, 5
toxic substances, 19
toy kitchens, 81
Tropical Smoothie, 213–14
tuna, 88
turkey
  Grub Worms and Dirt Bombs, 157–58
  Turkey, Cabbage, and Carrots over Rice,
    154
  Turkey Potpie, 152–53
type 2 diabetes, 66

Udi's (bread brand), 154

Van's nutrition bars, 154
vegetable gardens for kids, 81
vegetables
  Cajun Red Potato Fries, 166
  Candy-Cane Carrots, 177–78
  canned, 88
  Cinnamon-Spiced Sweet Potato, 167–68
  consumption of, in U.S., 165
  Cranberry Confetti Wild Rice, 171
  Cucumber Salad, 175
  frozen, 165
  Golden Beet Salad, 169–70
  Green Beans with Honey, 178
  Grilled Asparagus, 178–79
  Grilled Veggie Salad, 173–74
  guidelines for, 87
  and hyperactivity, 90
  Josh Prichard's Kickin' Vegan Potato
    Salad, 166–67
  Pocketknife Coleslaw, 171–72
  Rice Stuffing, 179

and rotation diet, 60
  South-of-the-Border Salad, 170
  Summer Festival Salad, 174–75
  Sweet Potato Fries, 168–69
  Toasted Quinoa Cran-Raisin Salad,
    172–73
vestibular system, weak, 39–40
vinaigrette recipe, 169–70
vinegars, 88
visual processing problems, 3–4, 6, 38–39
vitamin A, 90, 91, 94–95
vitamin B-1 (thiamine), 90, 91, 98–99
vitamin B-3 (niacin), 90, 91, 100
vitamin B-5 (pantothenic acid), 91, 100–101
vitamin B-6 (pyridoxine), 90, 97–98, 99
vitamin B-12, 13, 96–97, 99
vitamin C, 103–4
vitamin D, 90, 104–6
vitamin E, 106
vitamins, deficiencies in, 90
vomiting, 35, 42

walnuts: Cherry-Walnut Breakfast Loaf, 129
water, 60
wheat
  and addictions to foods, 17
  and elimination diet, 52
  and food labels, 63
  genetic modification of, 47
  and glycemic index (GI), 66
  and 10 Most Wanted List, 44
  See also gluten
Wheat Belly (Davis), 66
whole grains, 87, 90
withdrawal symptoms, 54
Woods, Collins, 140
wraps: Sweet Potato/Black Bean Burritos
    in Collard Wraps, 161–62

xanthan gum, 182

yeast infections, chronic, 67–68
yogurt, 68

zinc, 90, 91, 109
zucchinis
  Grilled Veggie Salad, 173–74
  Pureed Vegetable Soup with a Kick,
    133–34

ABOUT THE AUTHOR

Dr. Robert Melillo is a world-renowned chiropractic neurologist, professor, and researcher in child neurological disorders and creator of the Brain Balance Program. Since 1994 his program has helped thousands of children with autism spectrum disorder, ADHD, dyslexia, Tourette's syndrome, and other disorders. His Brain Balance Achievement Centers are located throughout the United States. Dr. Melillo lives in Rockville Centre, New York, with his wife and three children. Visit brainbalancecenters.com.